I0419634

Published by
Nature Photobook Publishing

- African Crane
- American Goldfinch
- Bald Eagle
- Black Capped Chickadee
- Blue Jay
- Budgie
- Canadian Goose
- Chicken
- Duckling
- Falcon
- Flamingo
- Grey Heron
- Hawk
- Hummingbird
- Kingfisher
- Lesser Swamp Warbler
- Macaw
- Mallard Duck
- Mourning Dove
- Northern Cardinal
- Oriole
- Osprey
- Ostrich
- Owl
- Peacock
- Pelican
- Penguin
- Pigeon
- Puffin
- River Tern
- Robin
- Seagull
- Siskin
- Snowy Egret
- Sparrow
- Swan
- Toucan
- Wild Goose
- Woodpecker
- Wren

African Crane

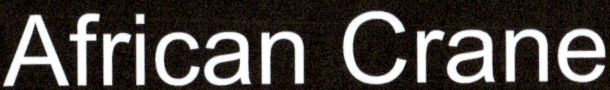

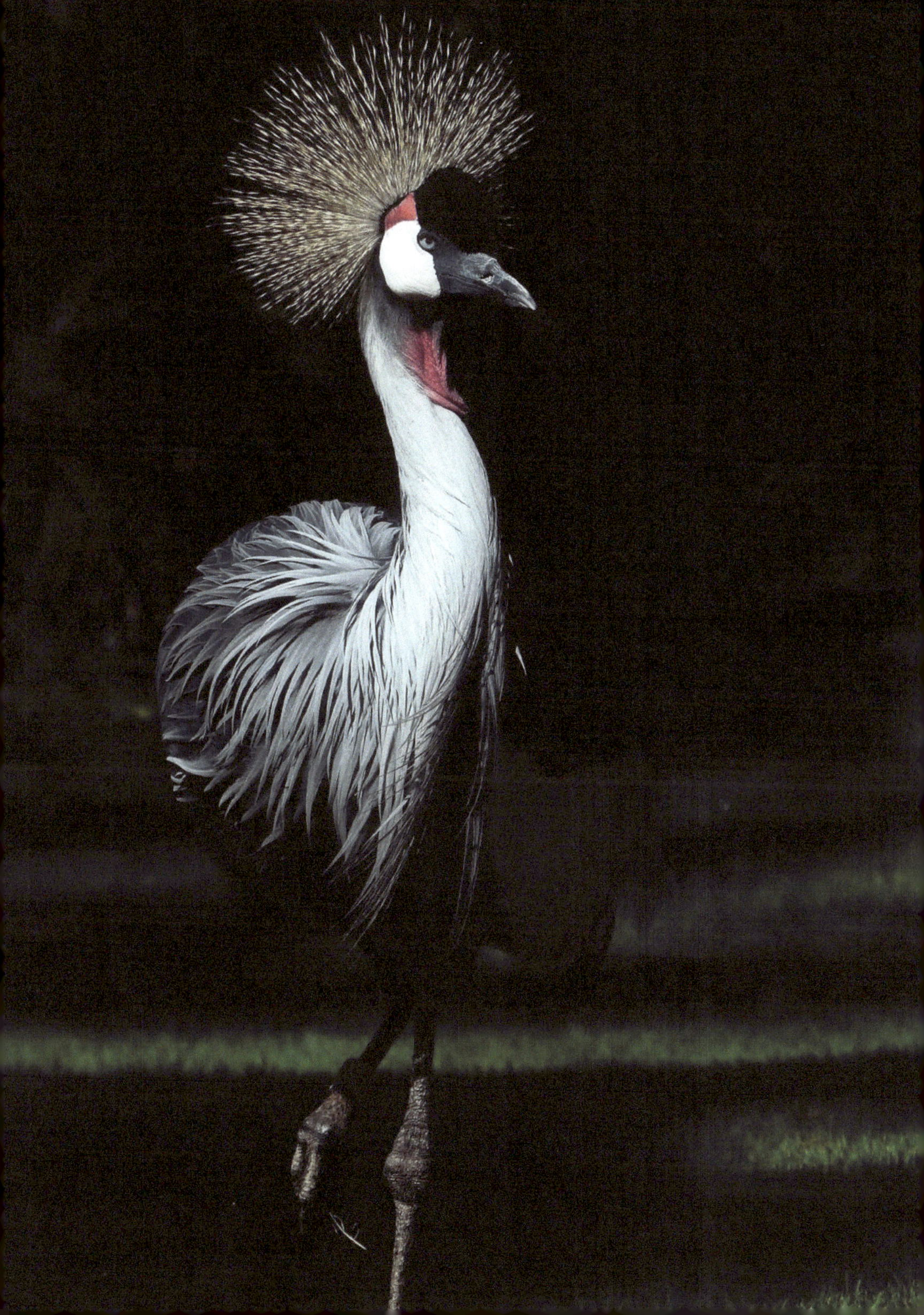

American Goldfinch

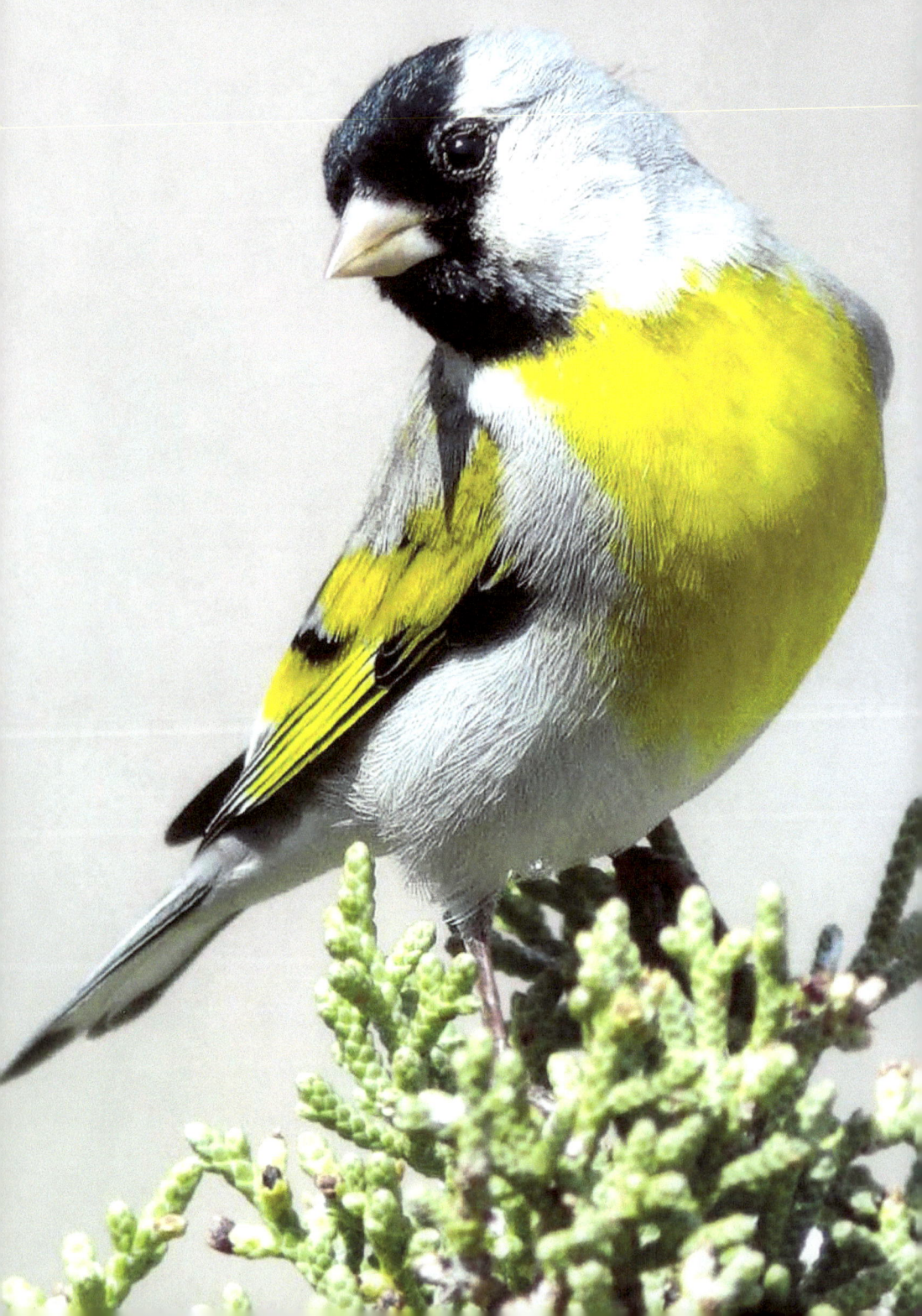

Bald Eagle

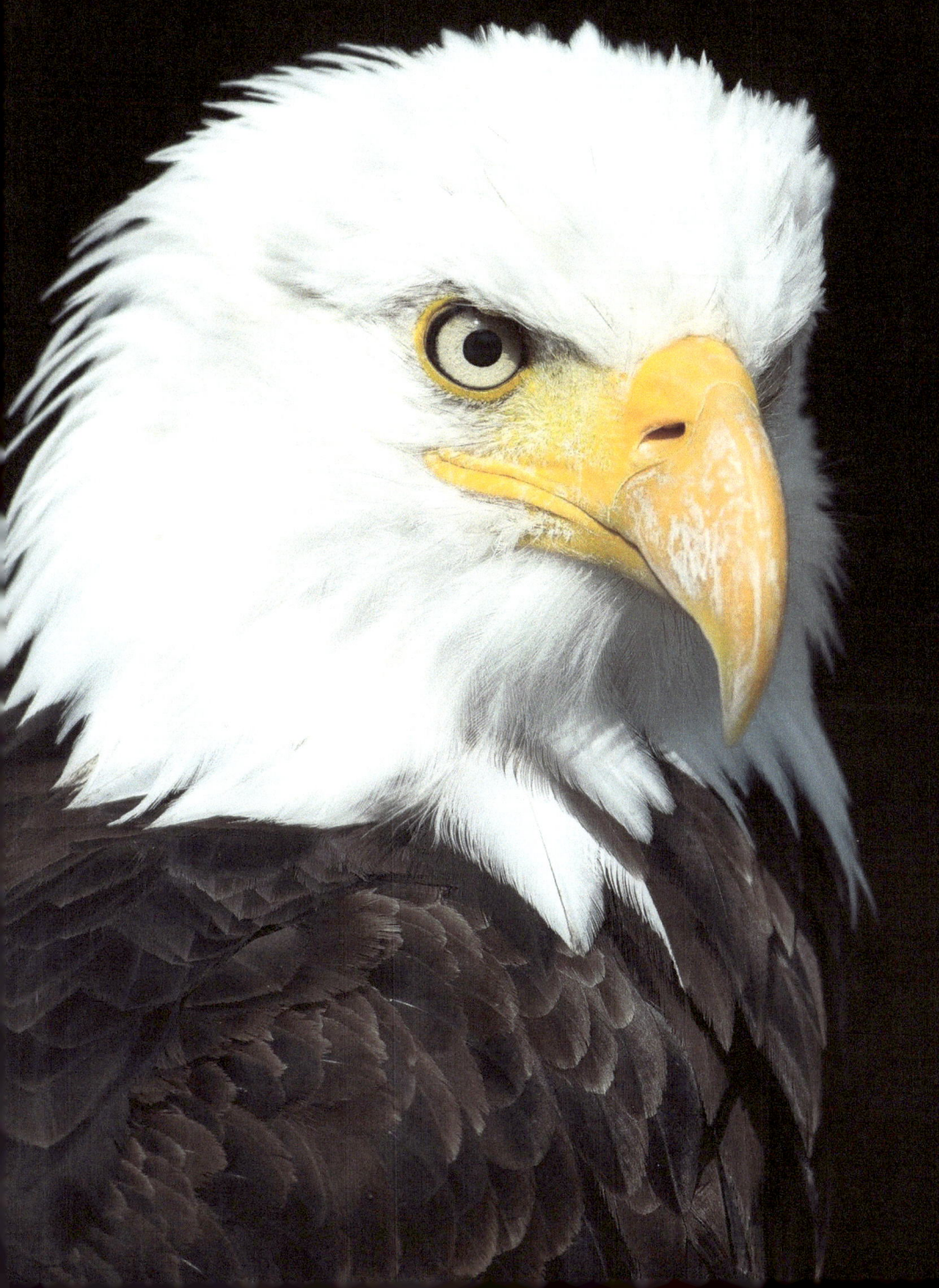

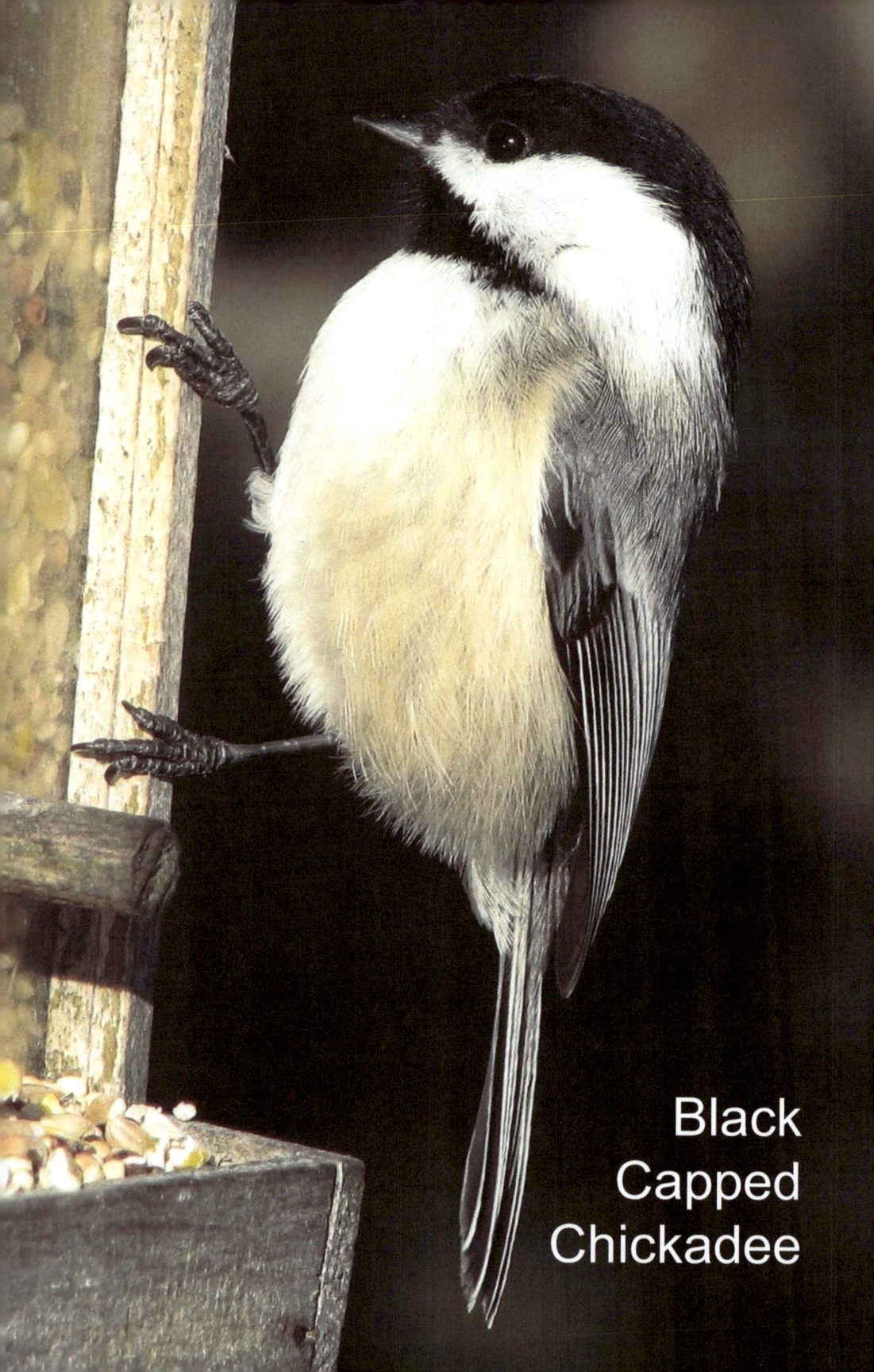

Black
Capped
Chickadee

Blue Jay

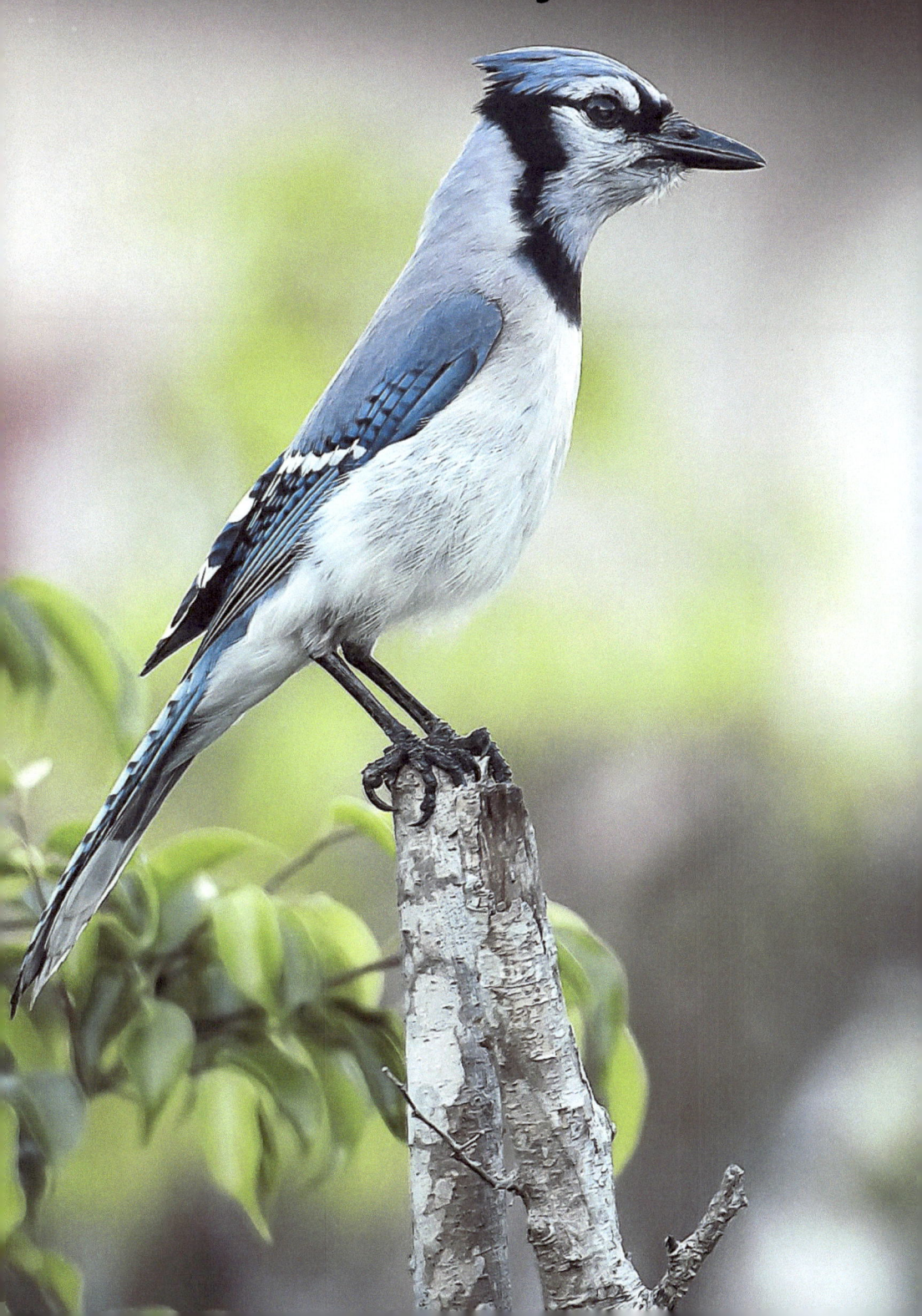

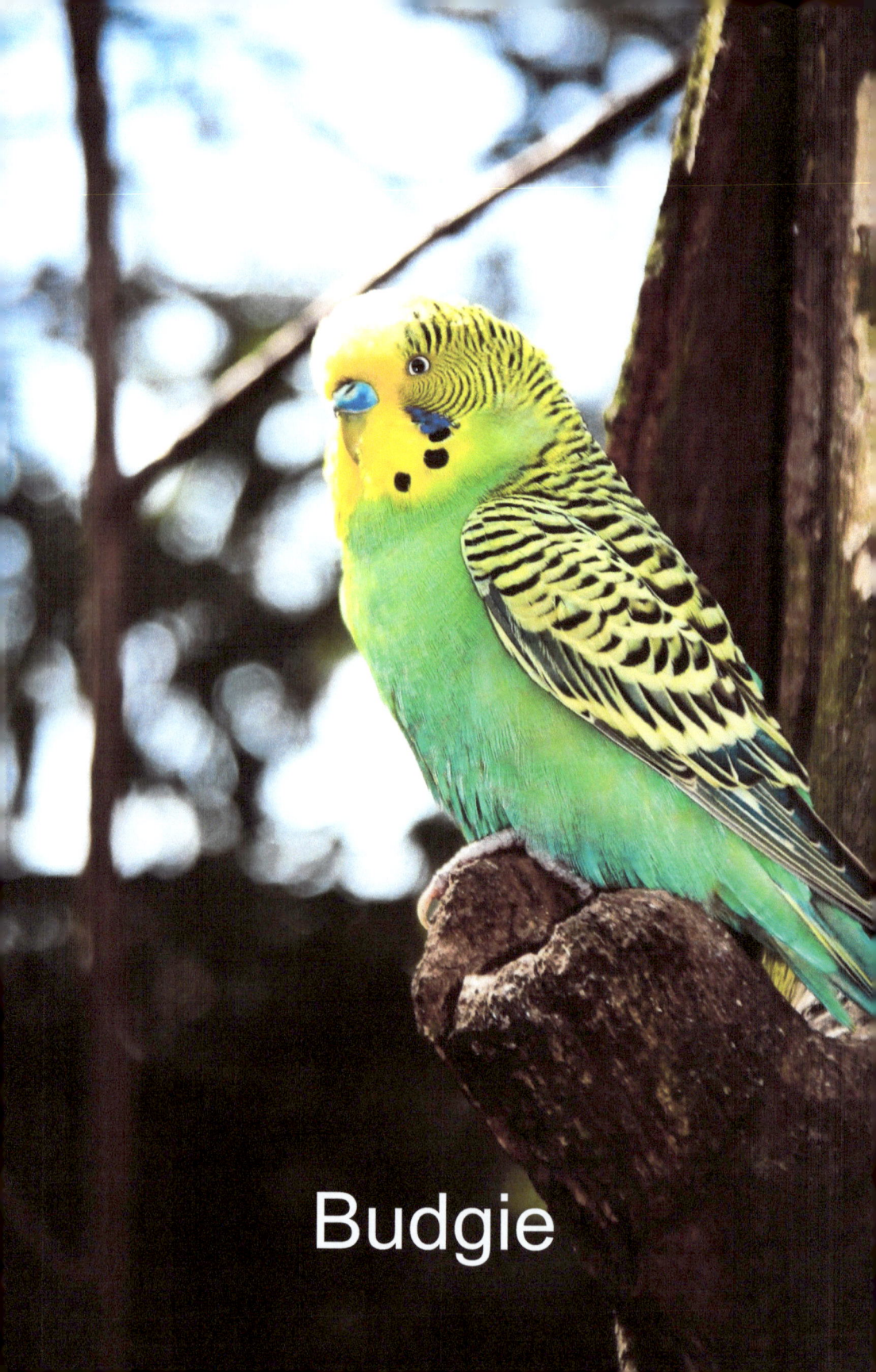

Budgie

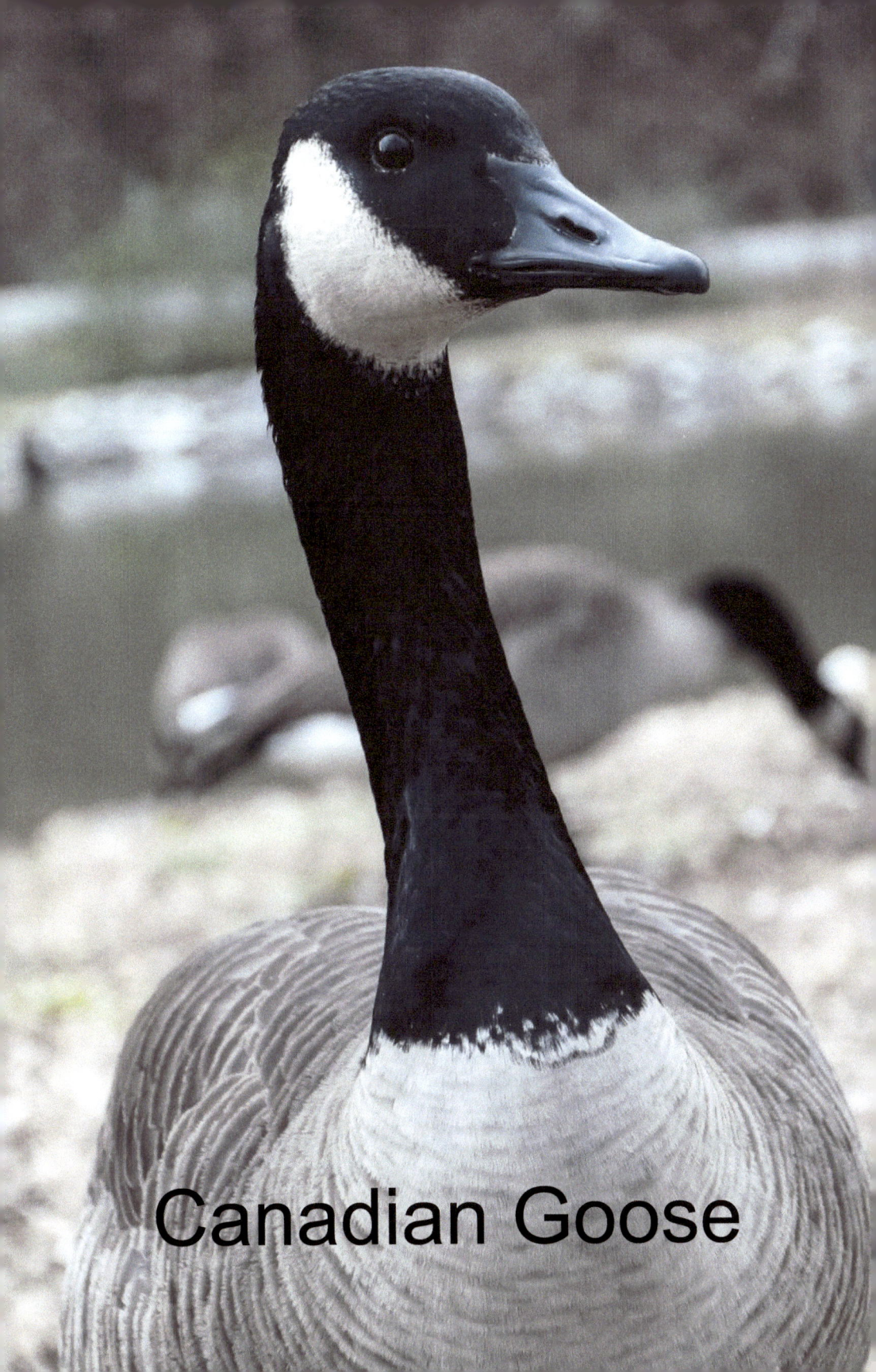

Canadian Goose

Chicken

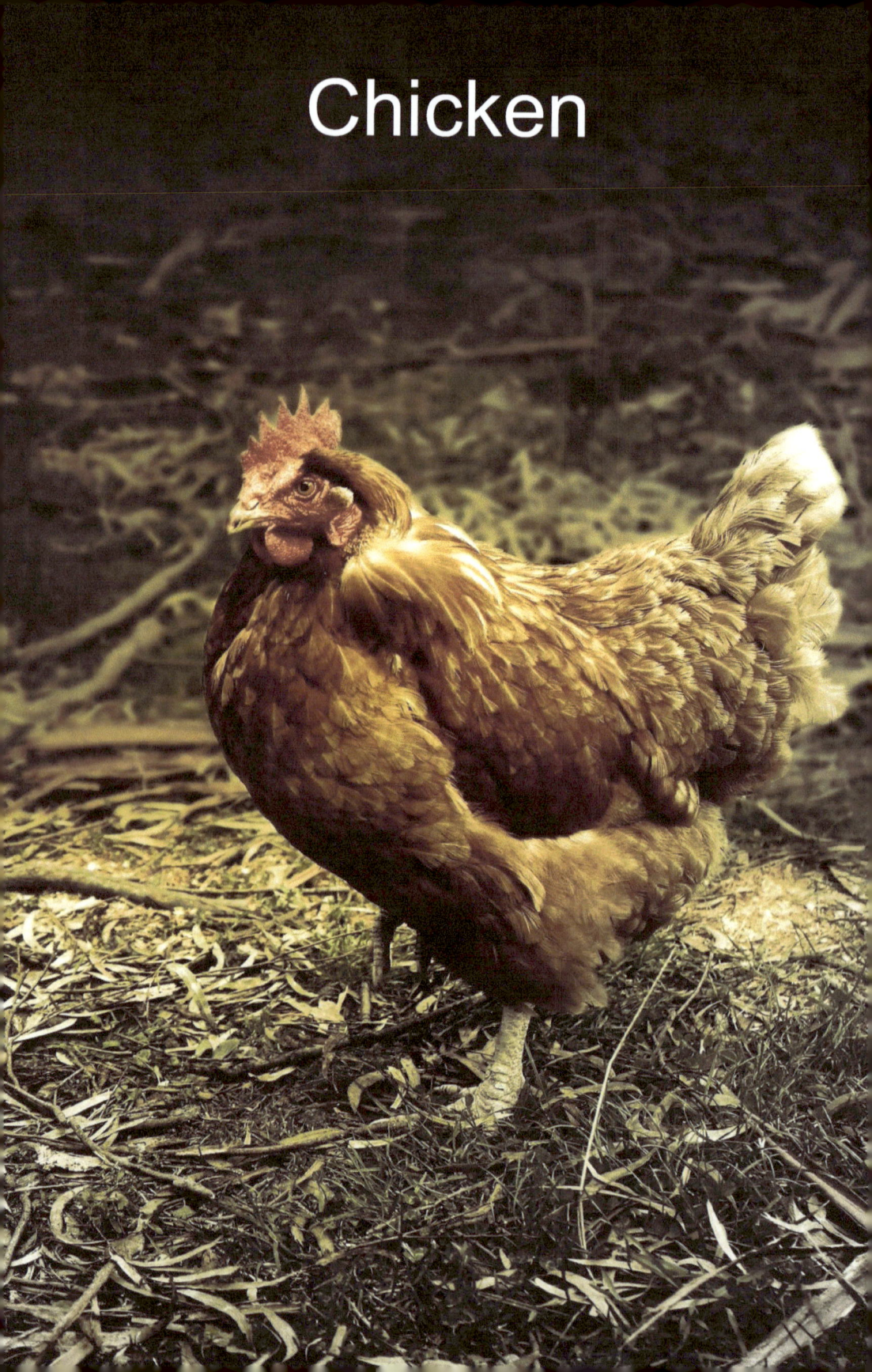

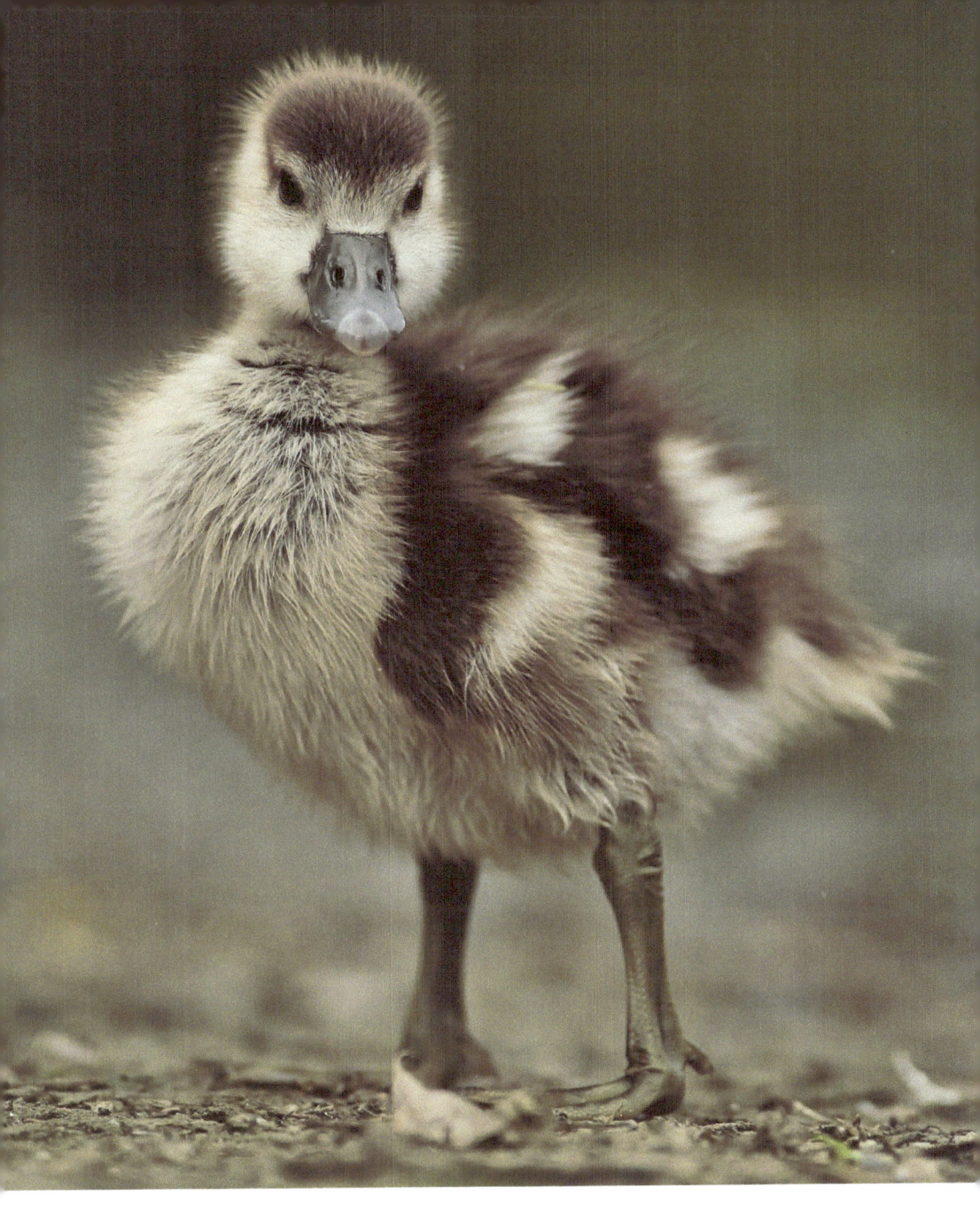

Duckling

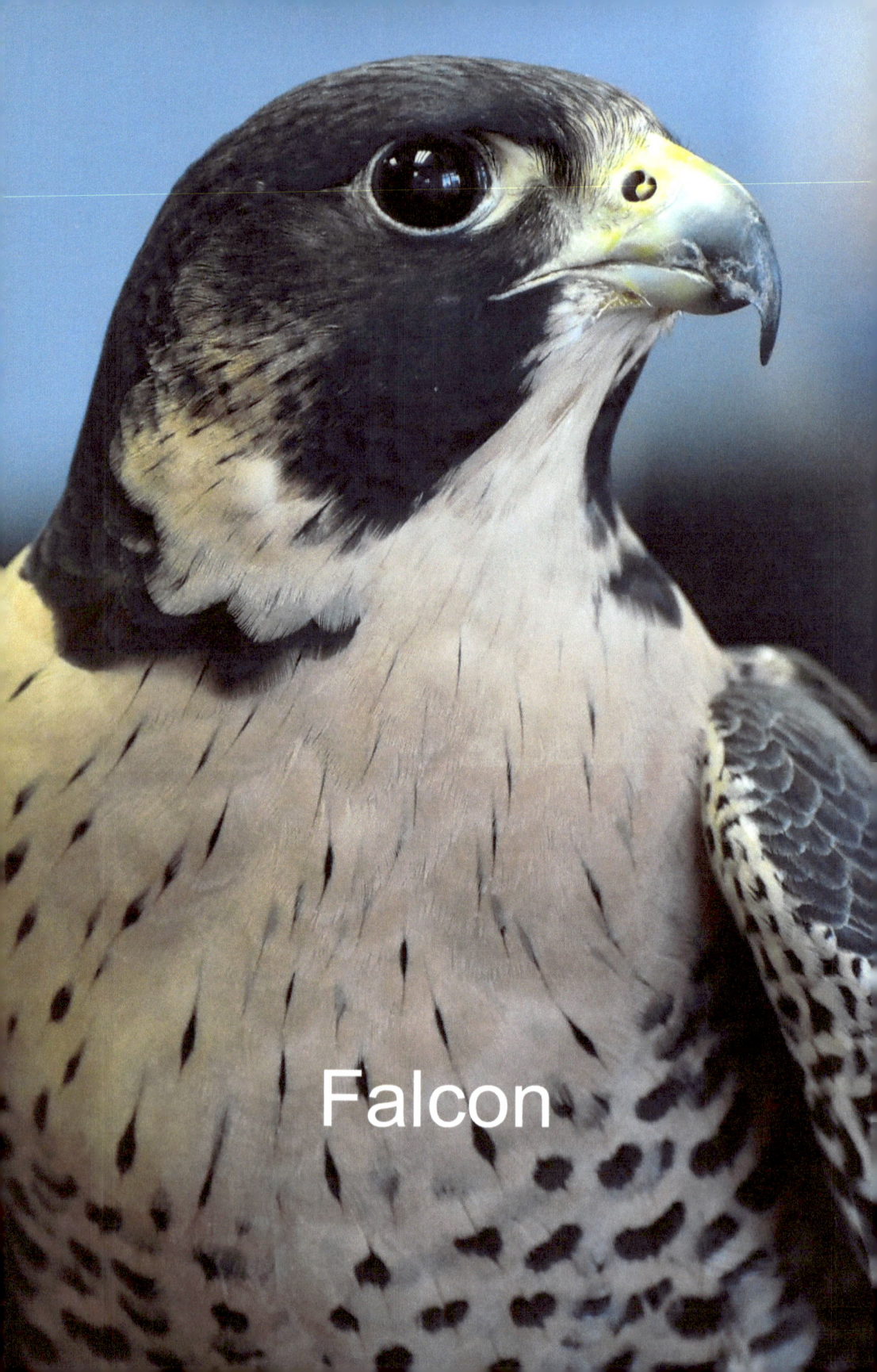

Falcon

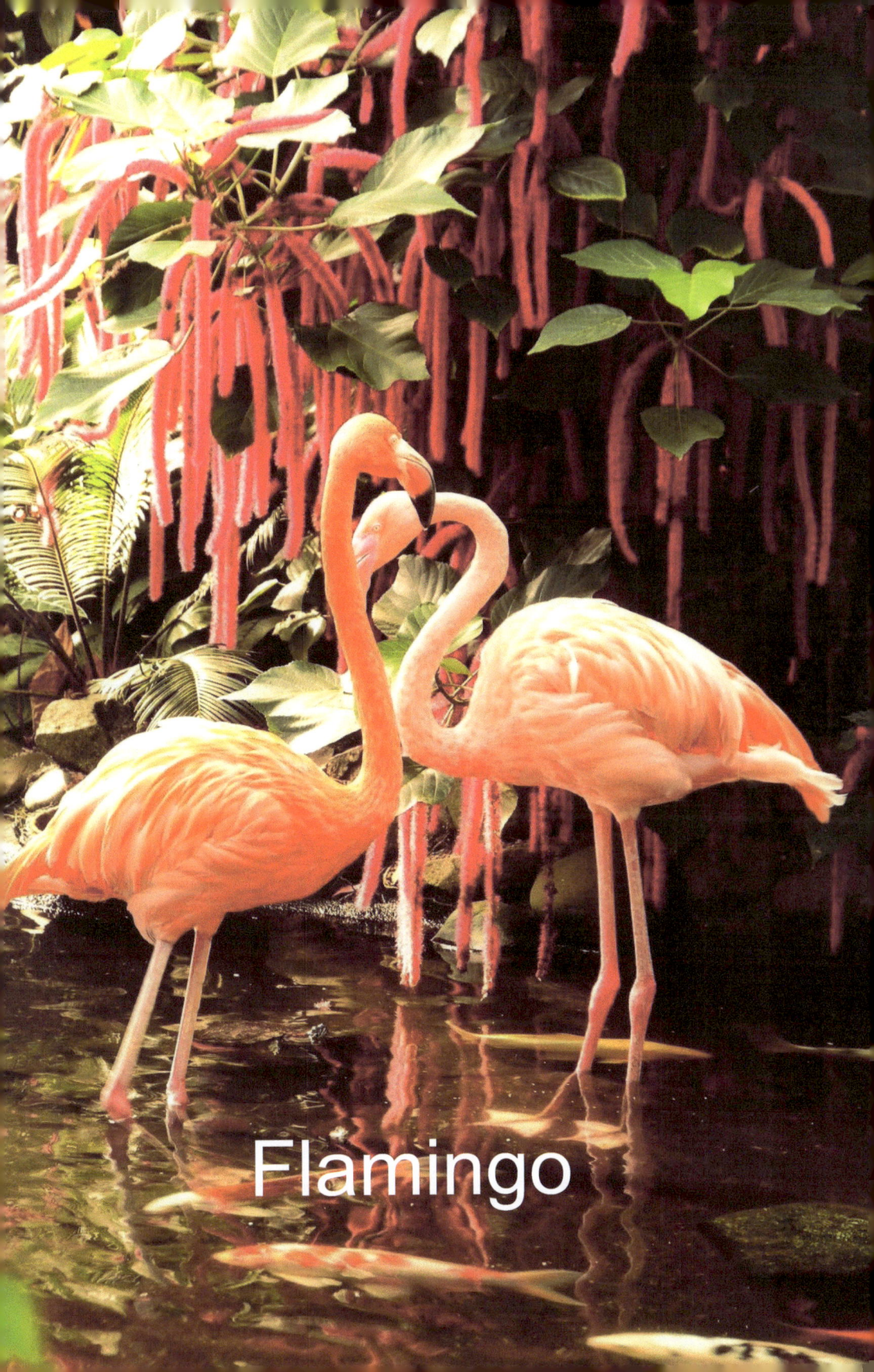

Flamingo

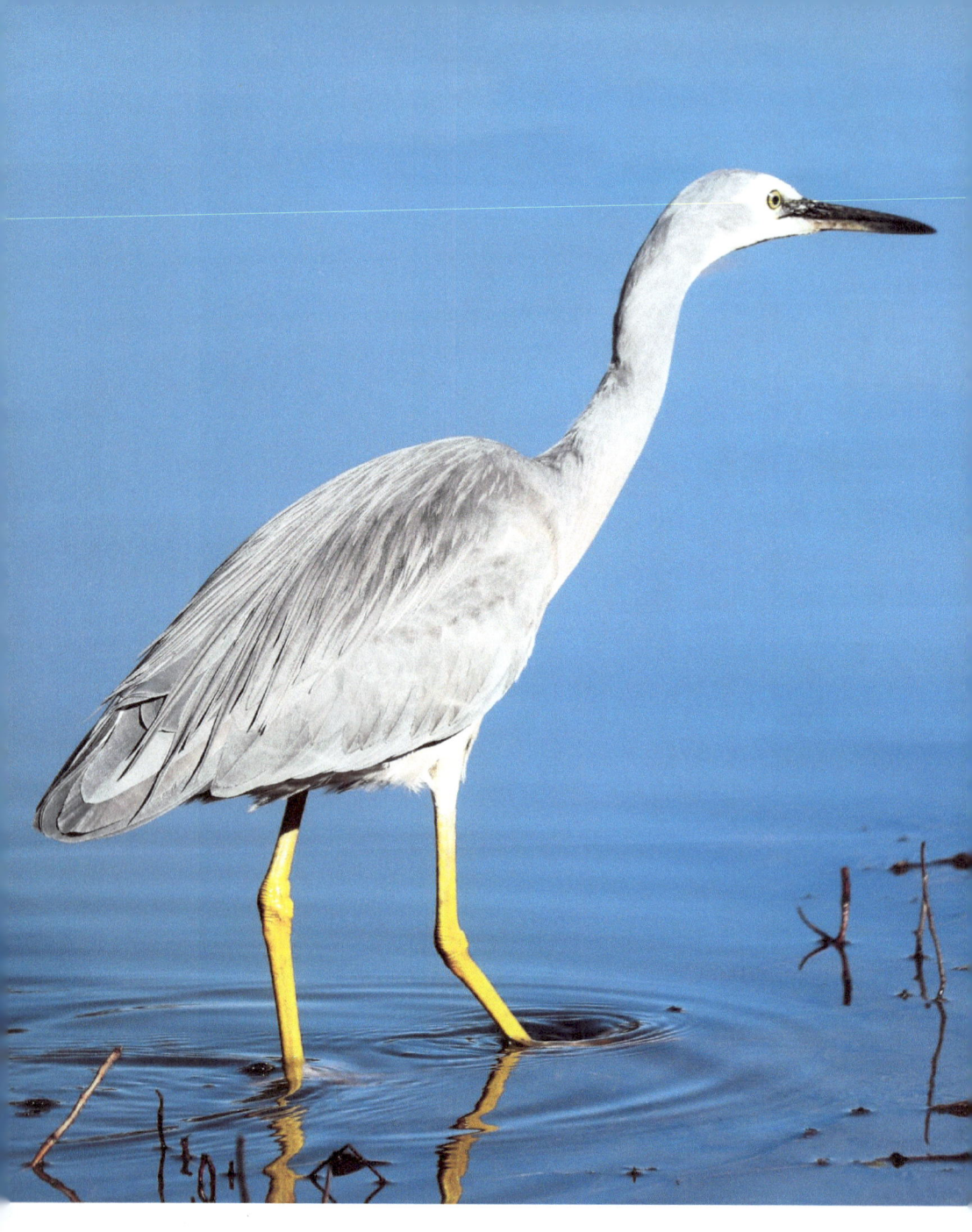

Grey Heron

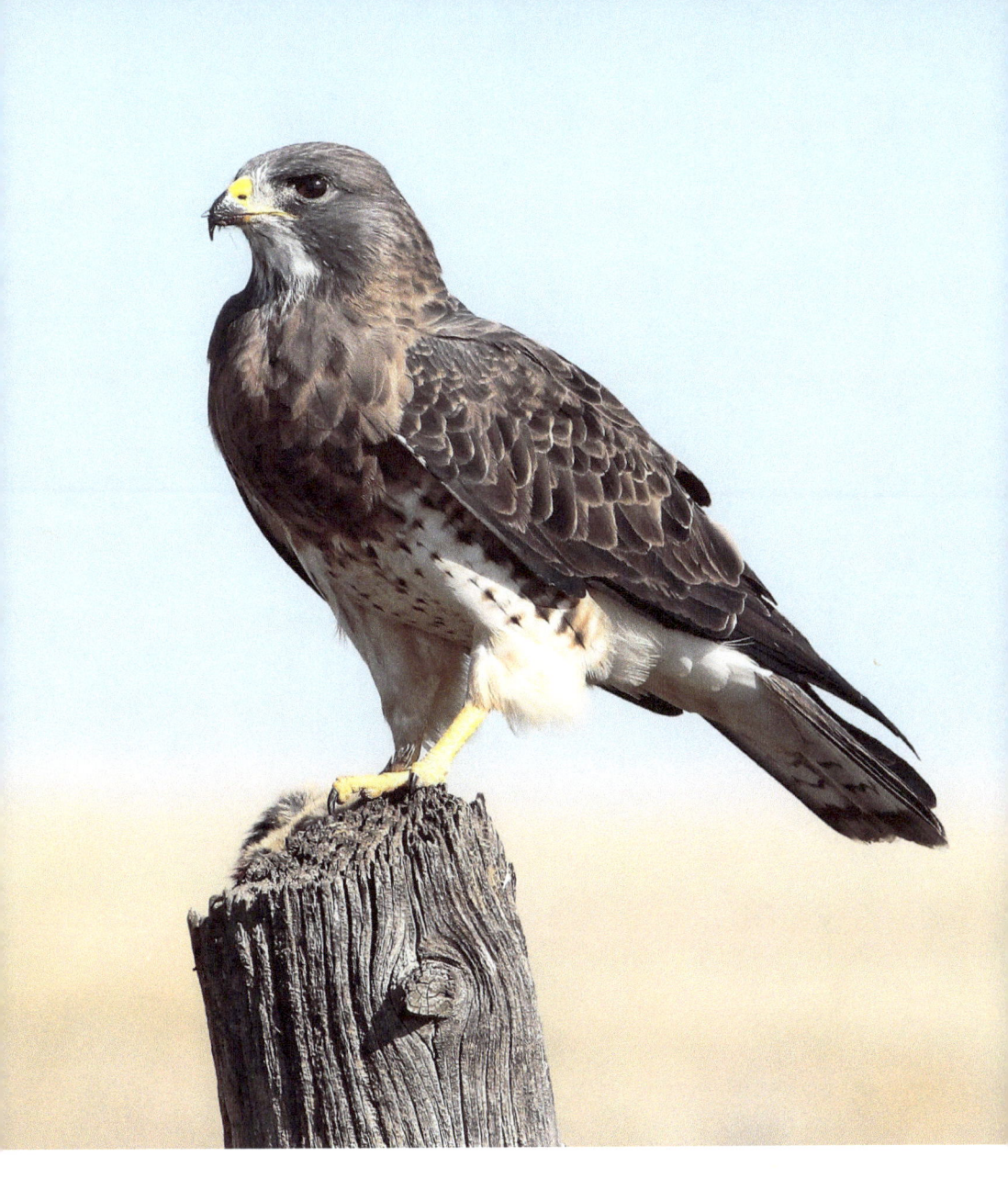

Hawk

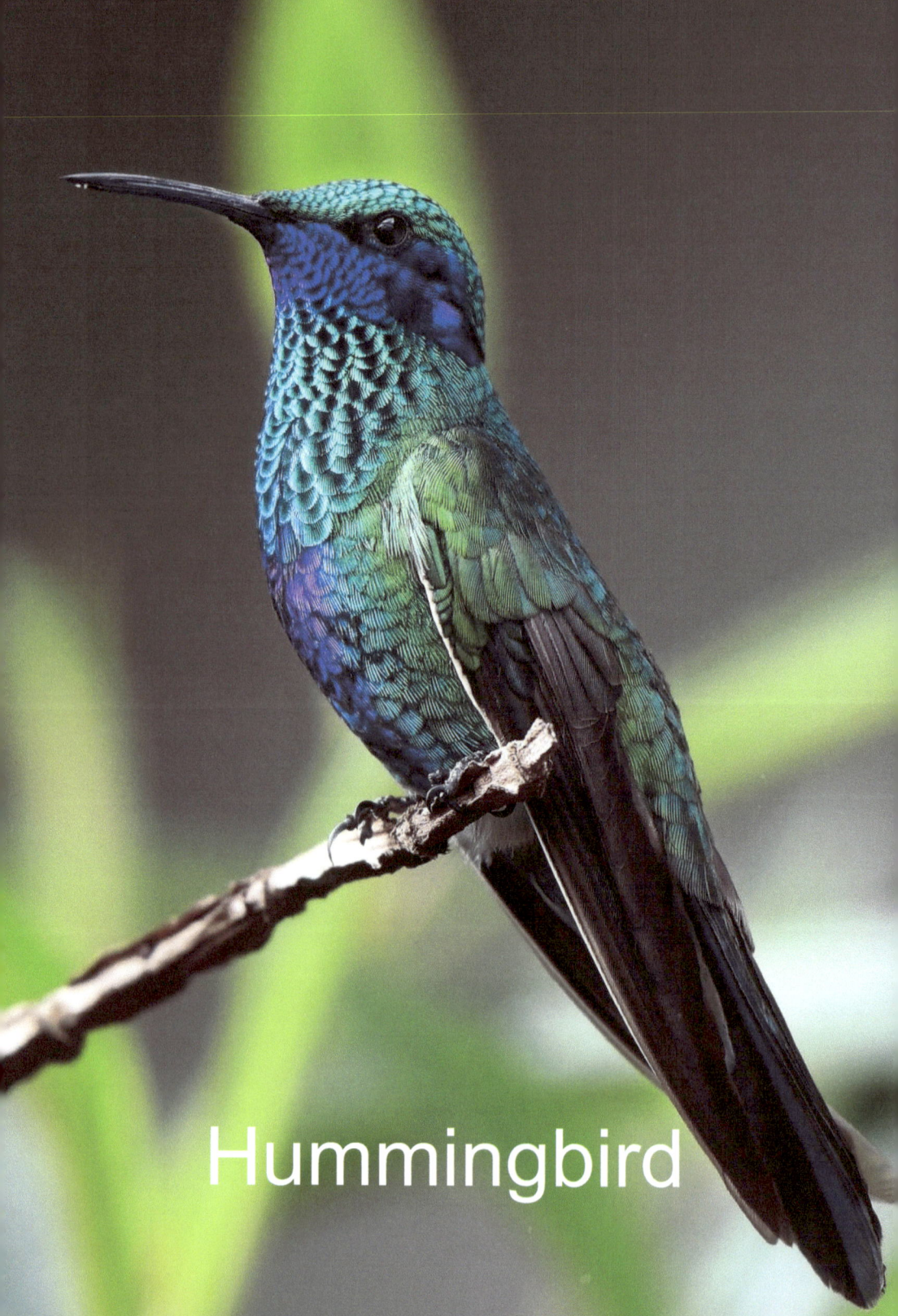

Hummingbird

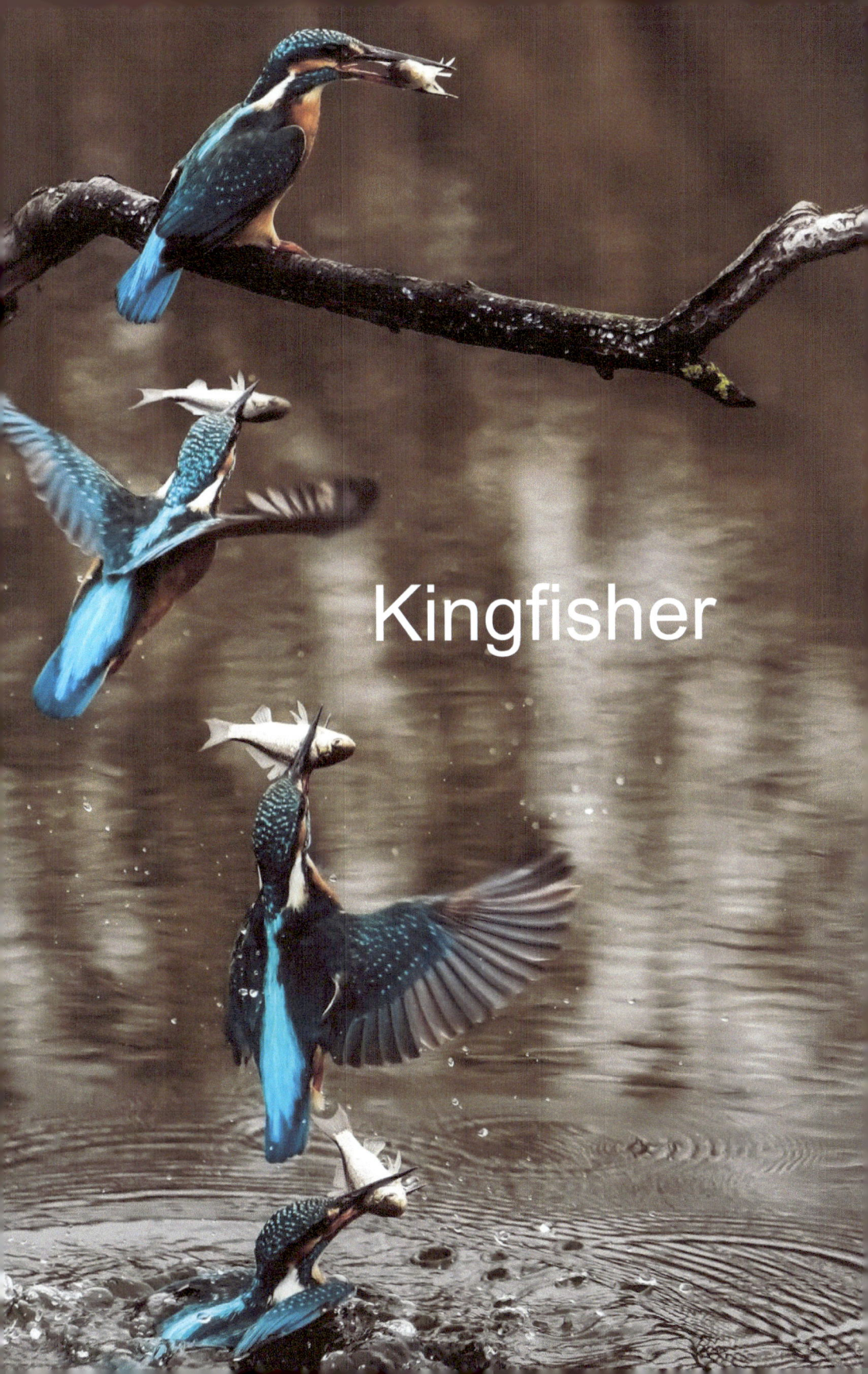

Kingfisher

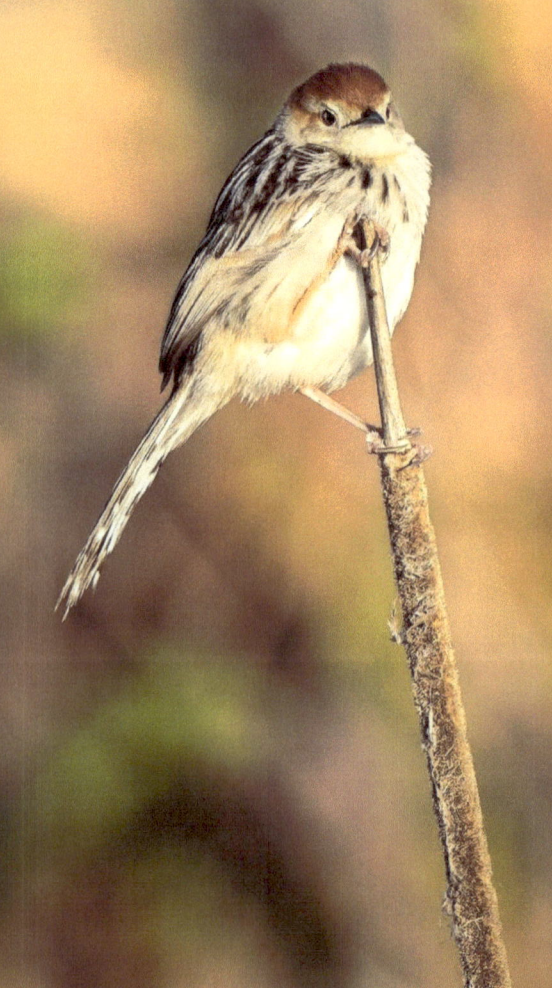

Lesser Swamp Warbler

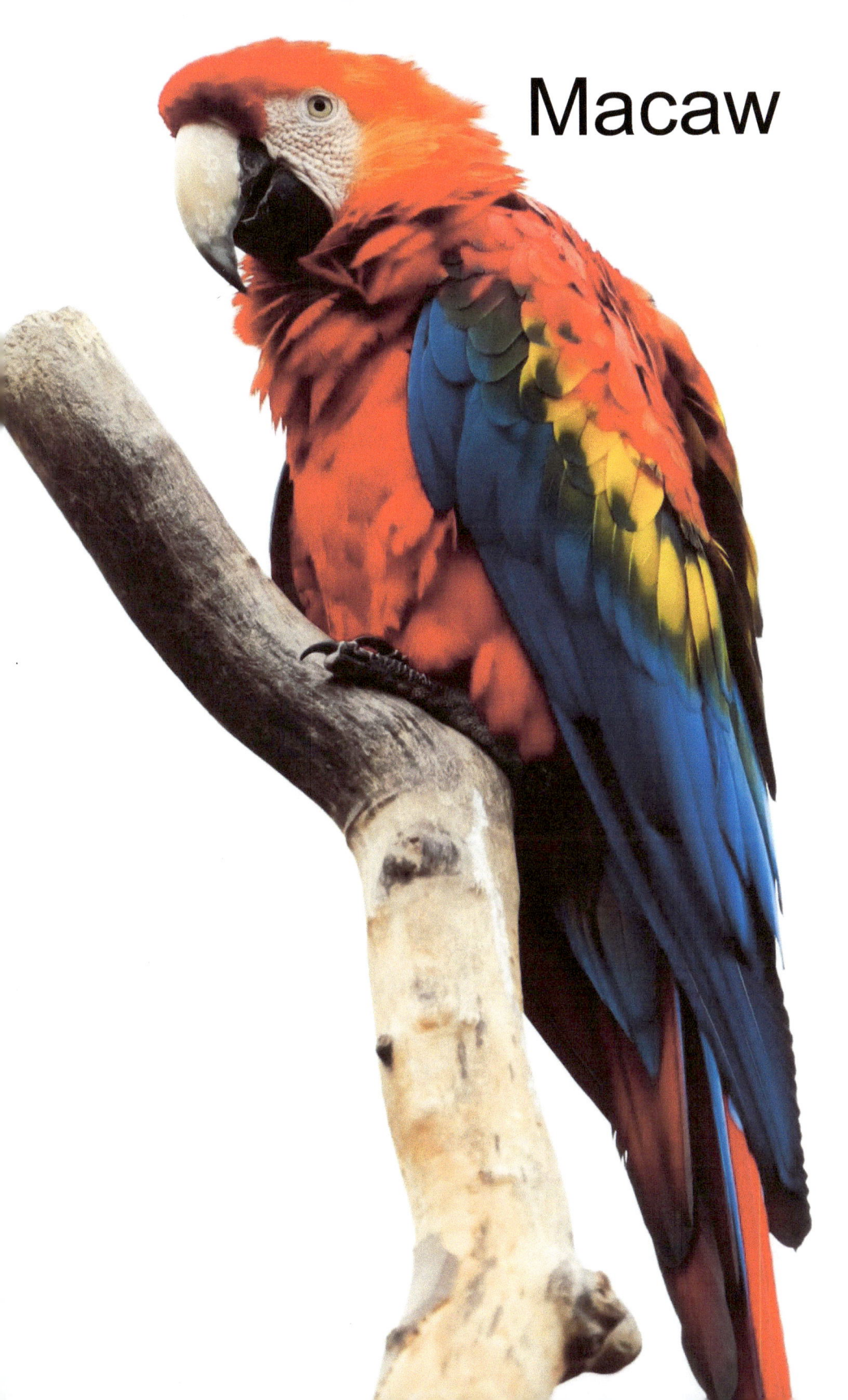

Macaw

Mallard Duck

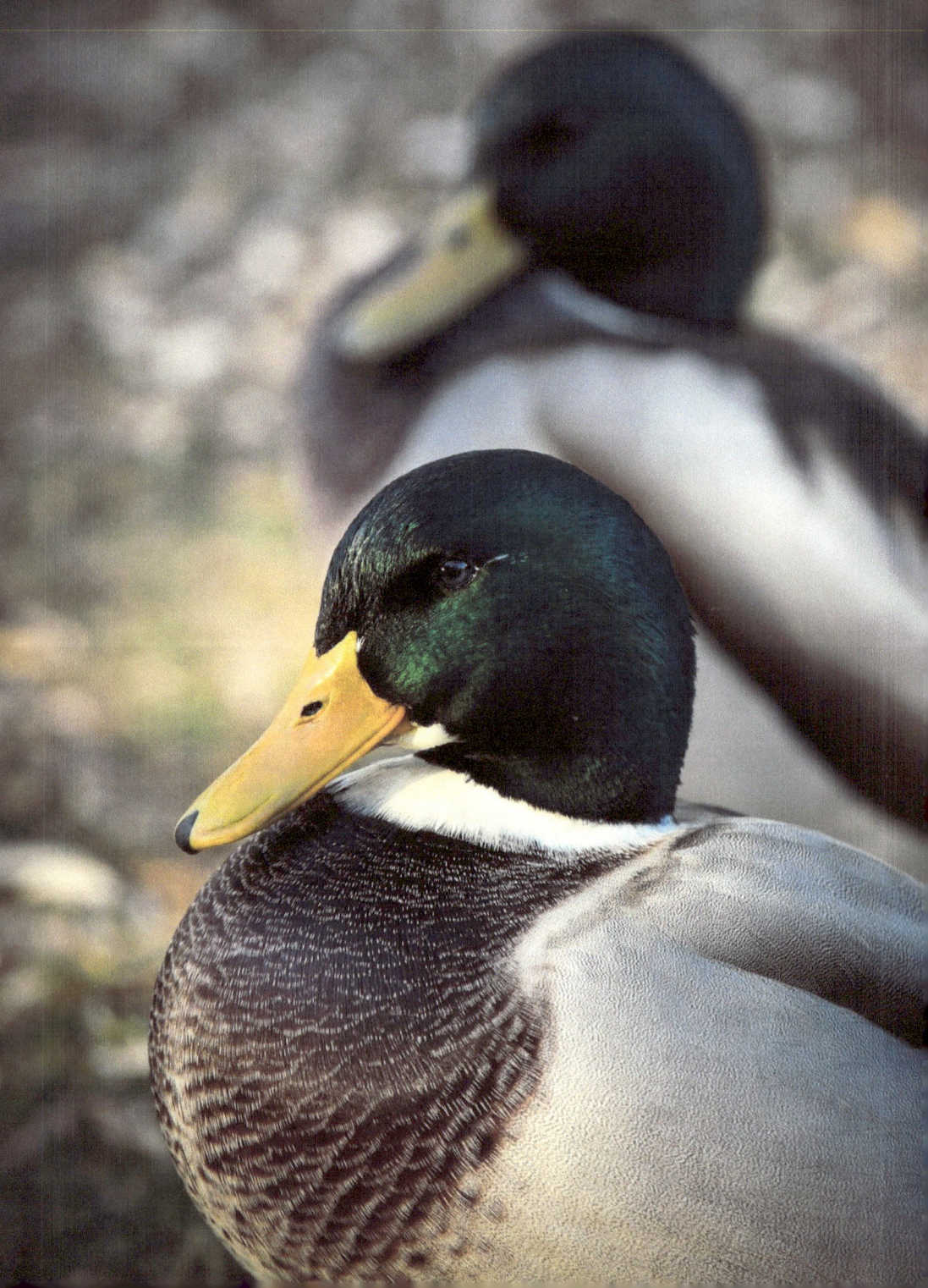

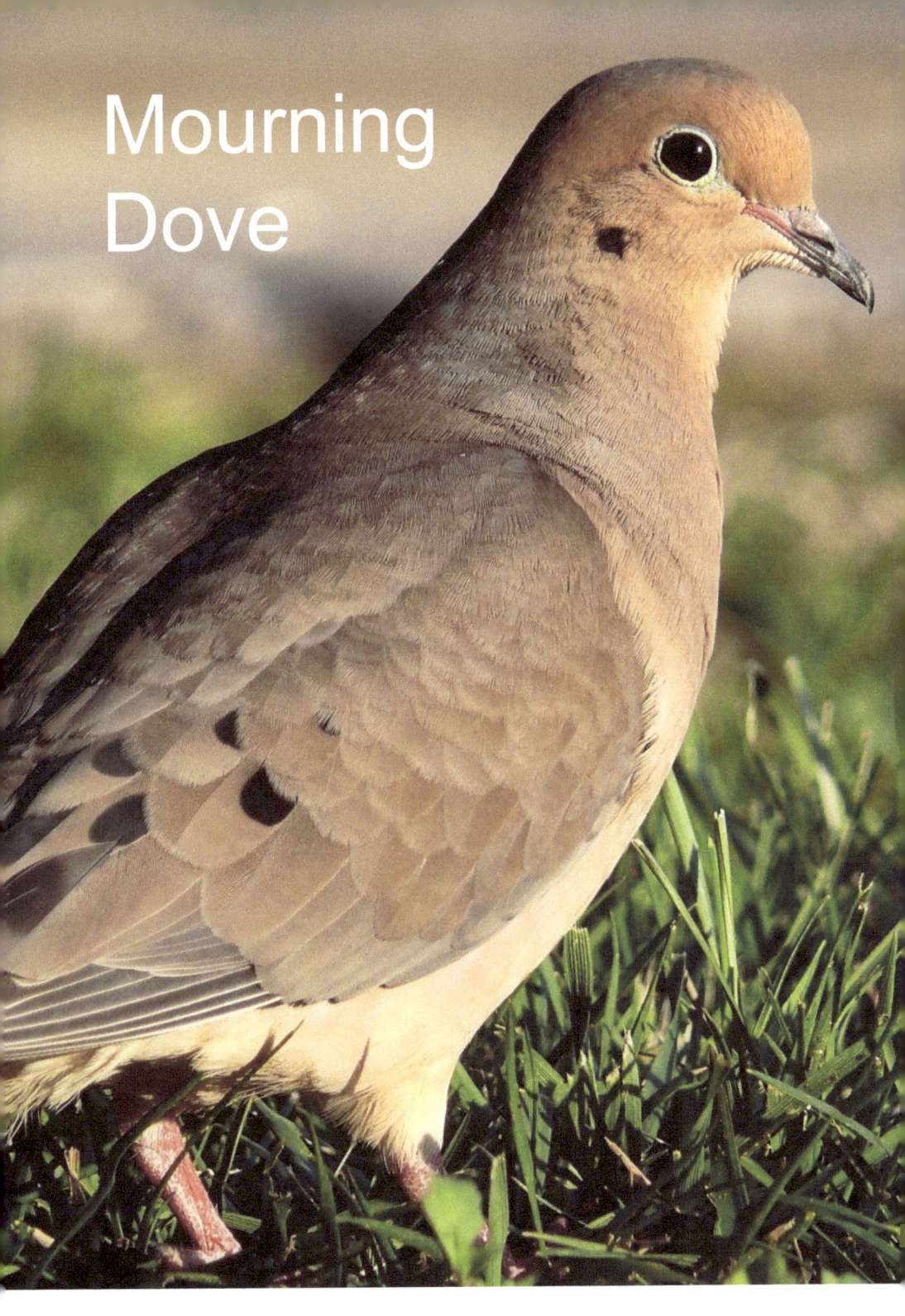

Mourning Dove

Northern Cardinal

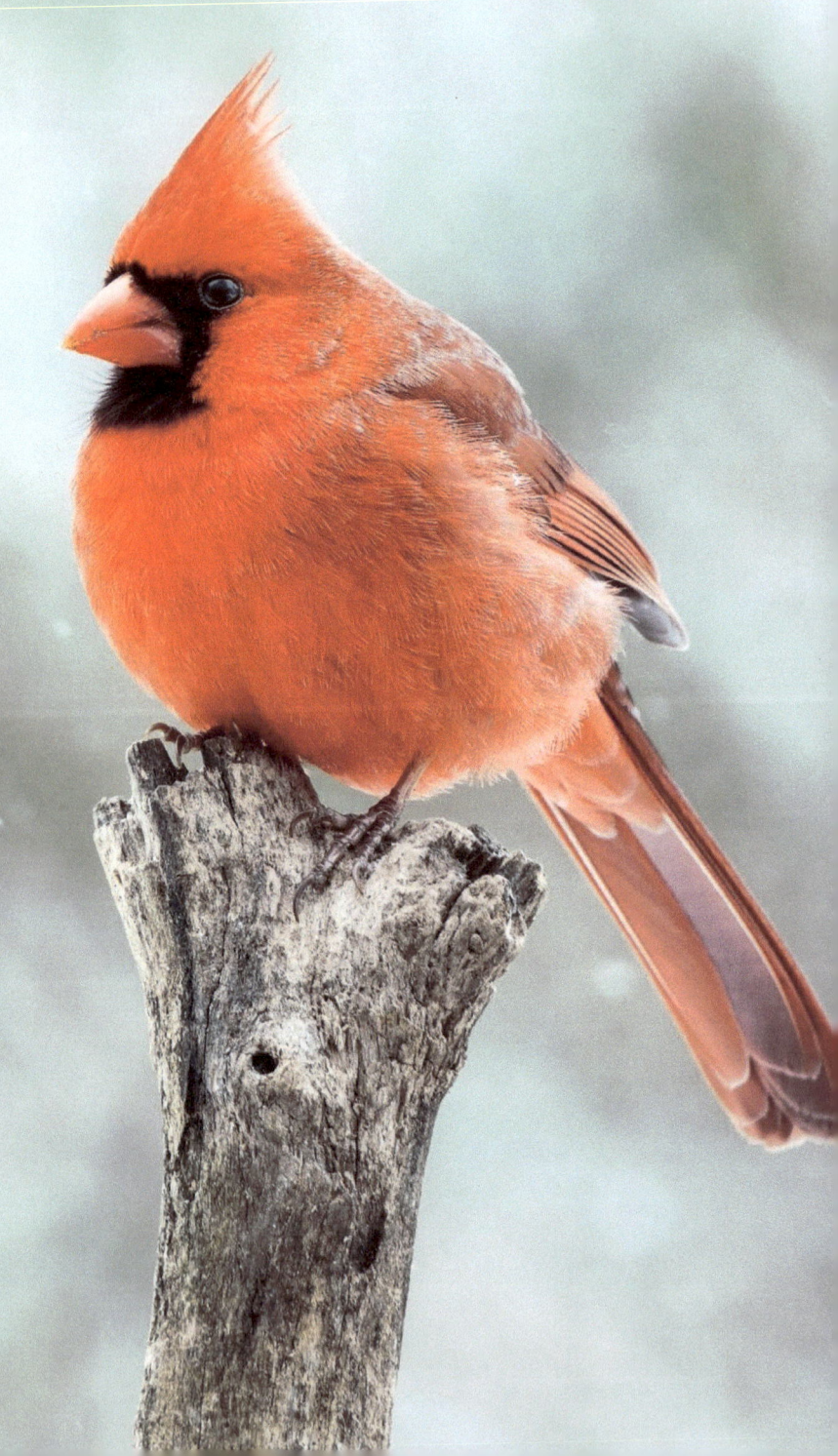

Oriole

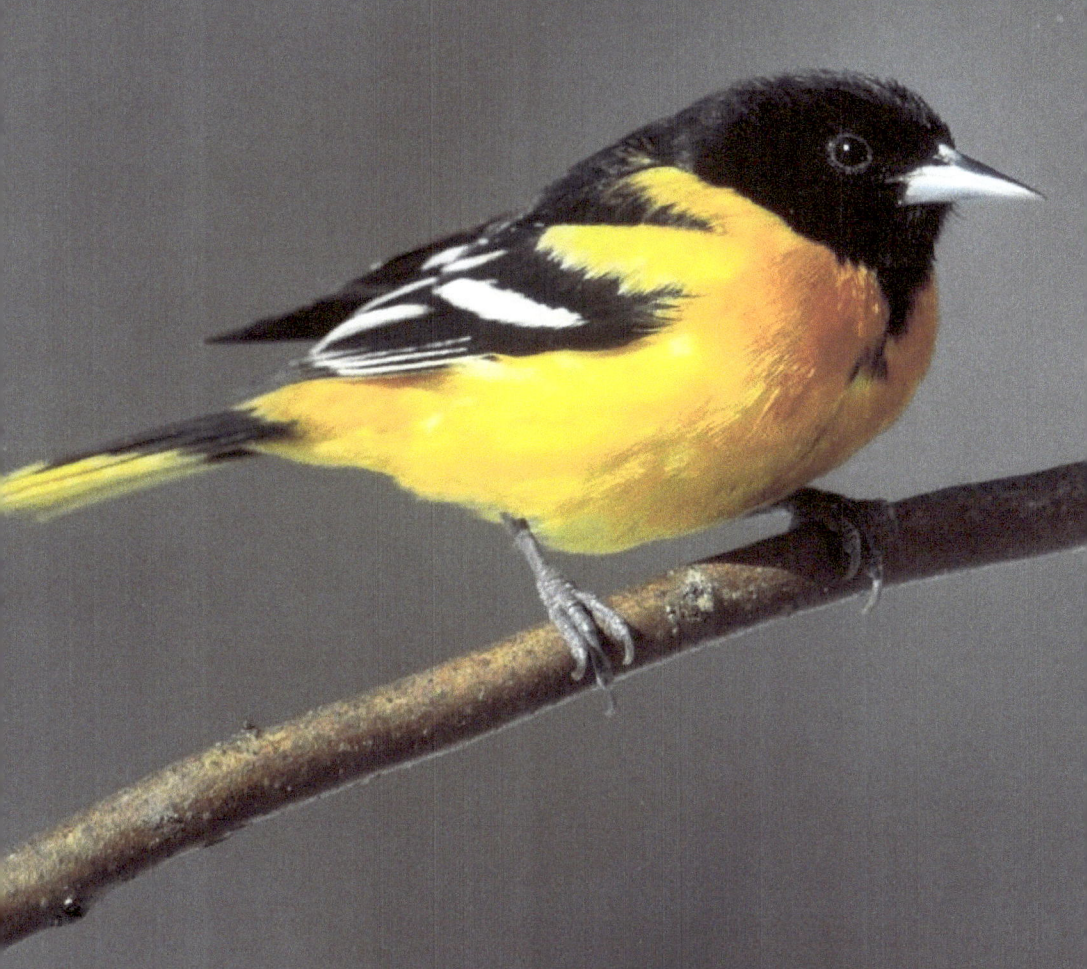

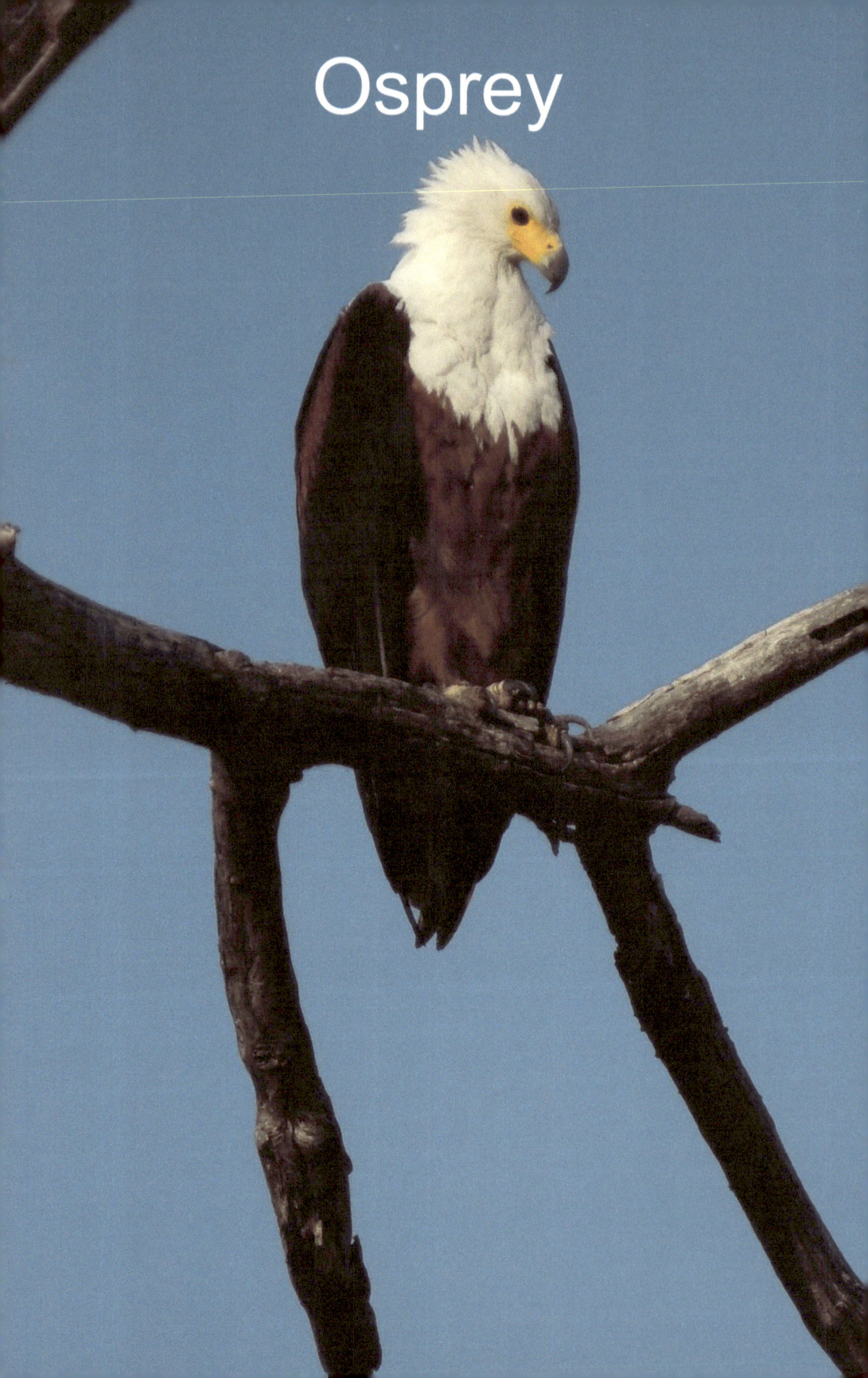

Osprey

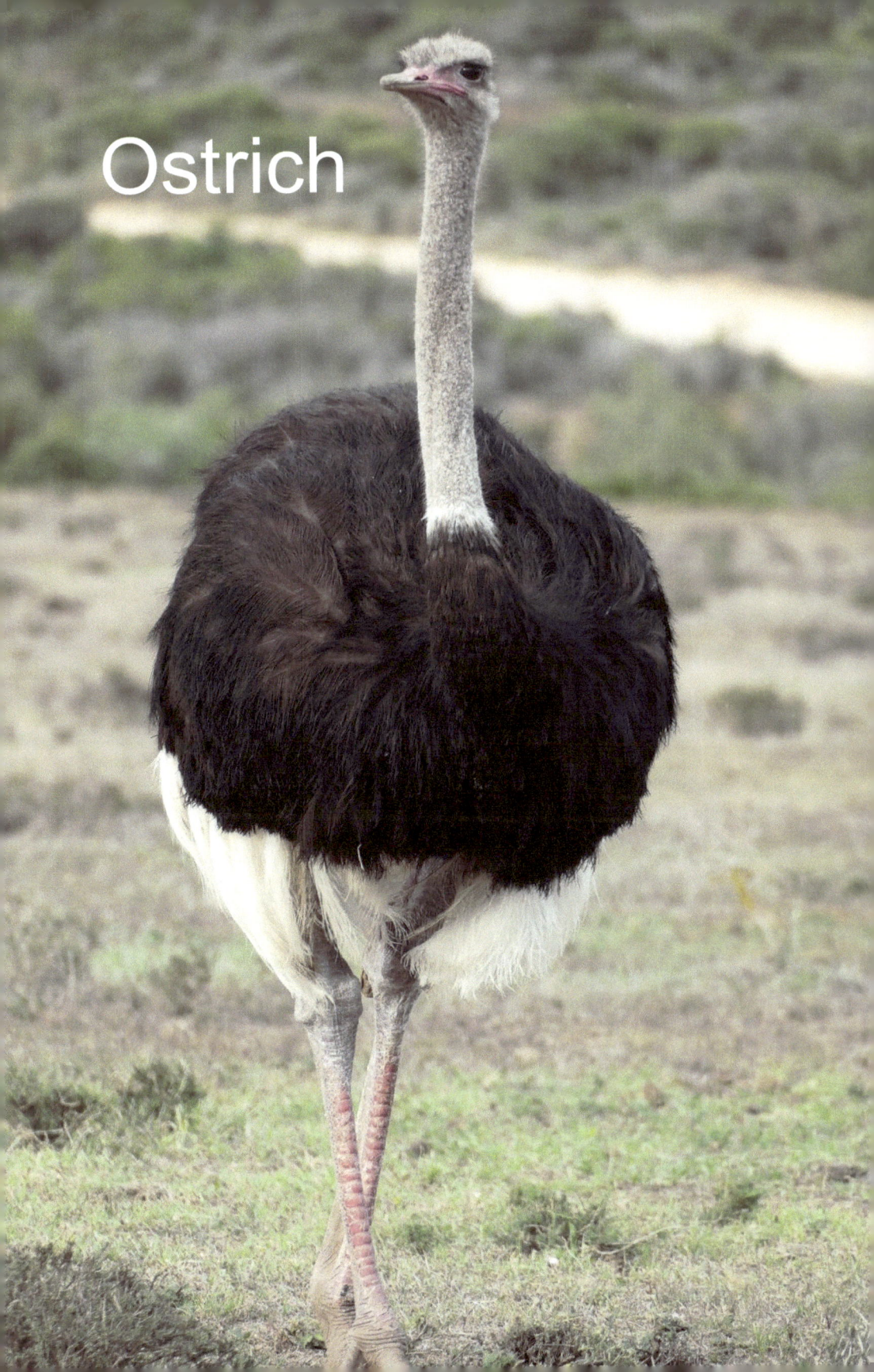

Ostrich

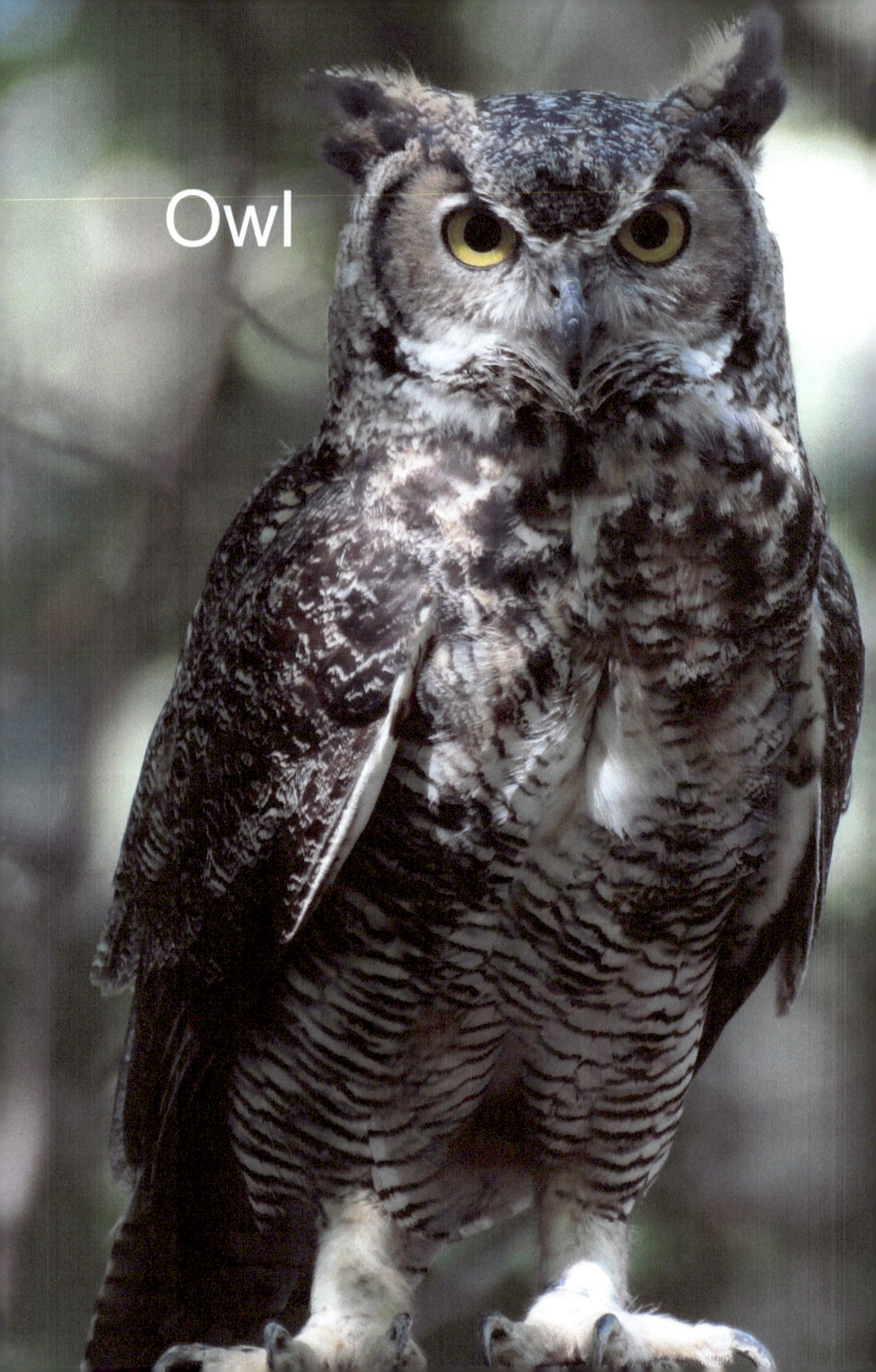

Owl

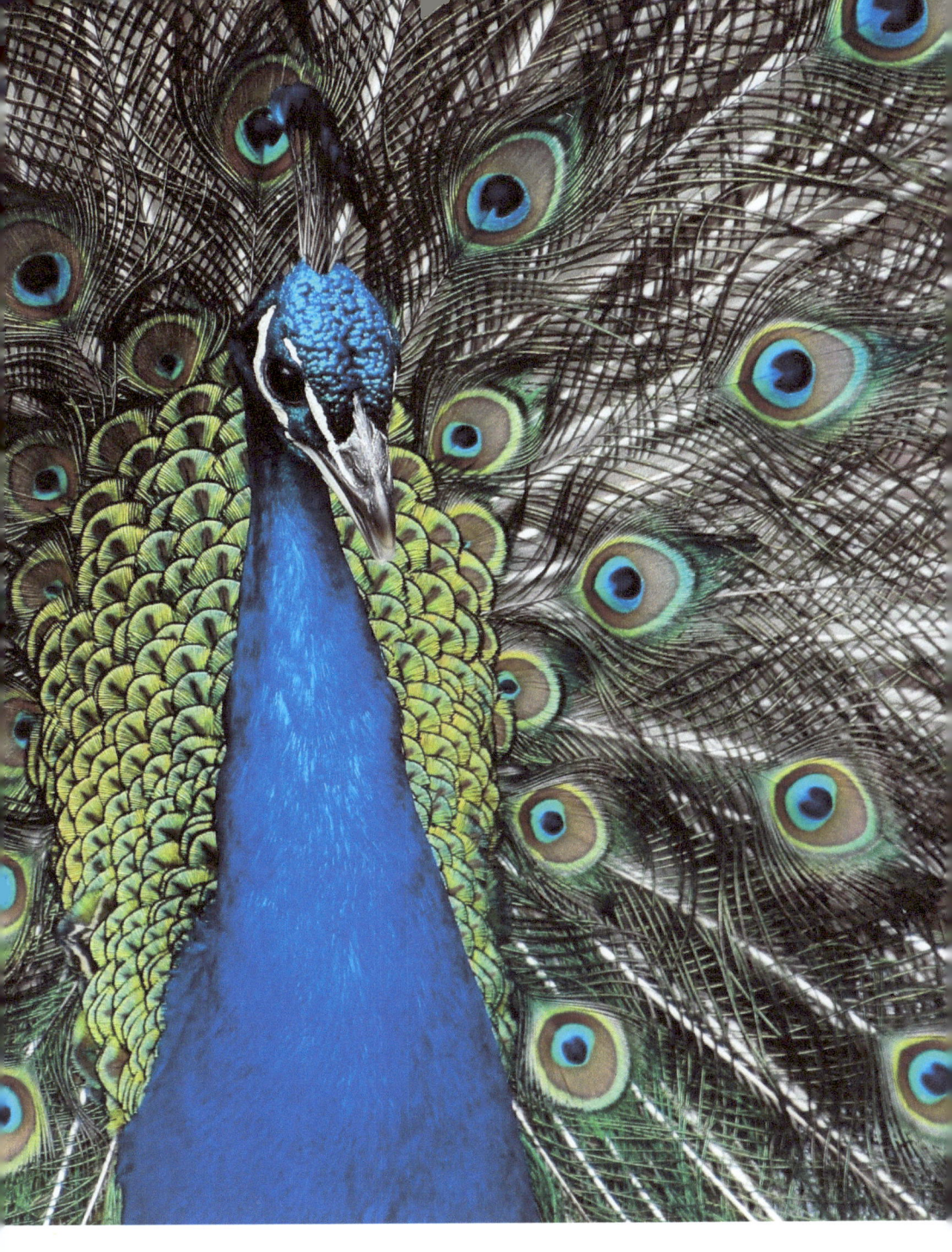

Peacock

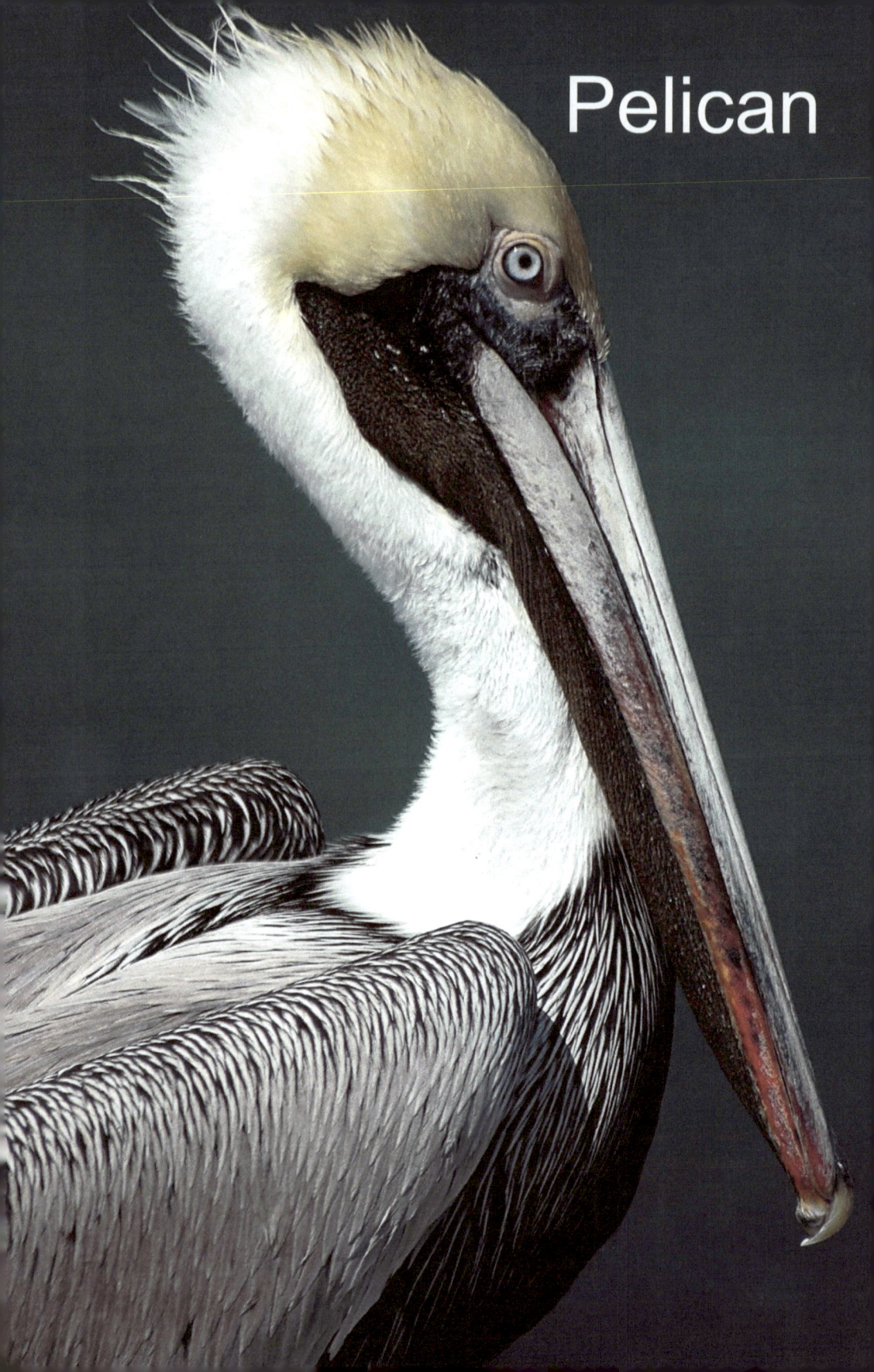

Pelican

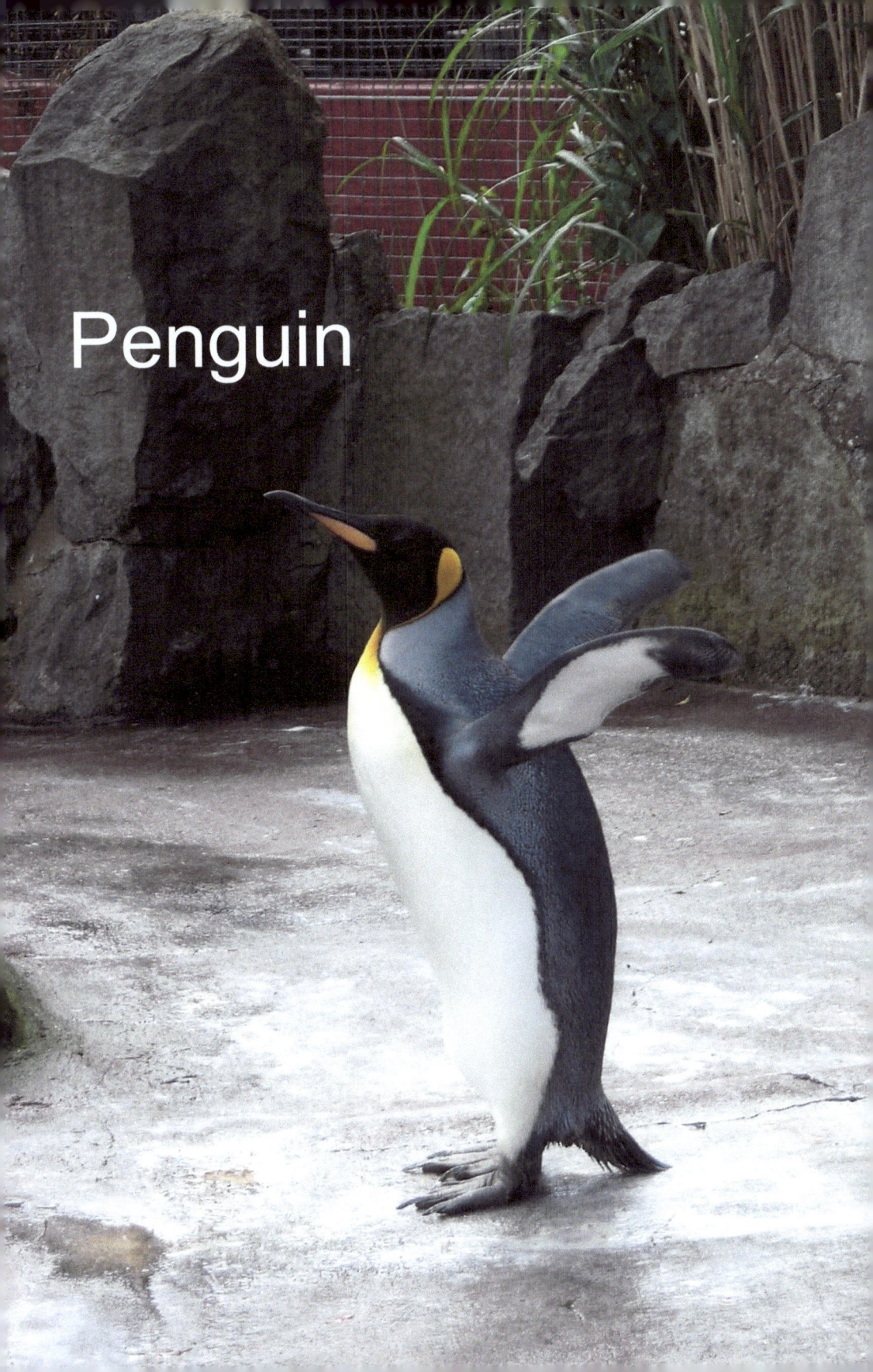

Penguin

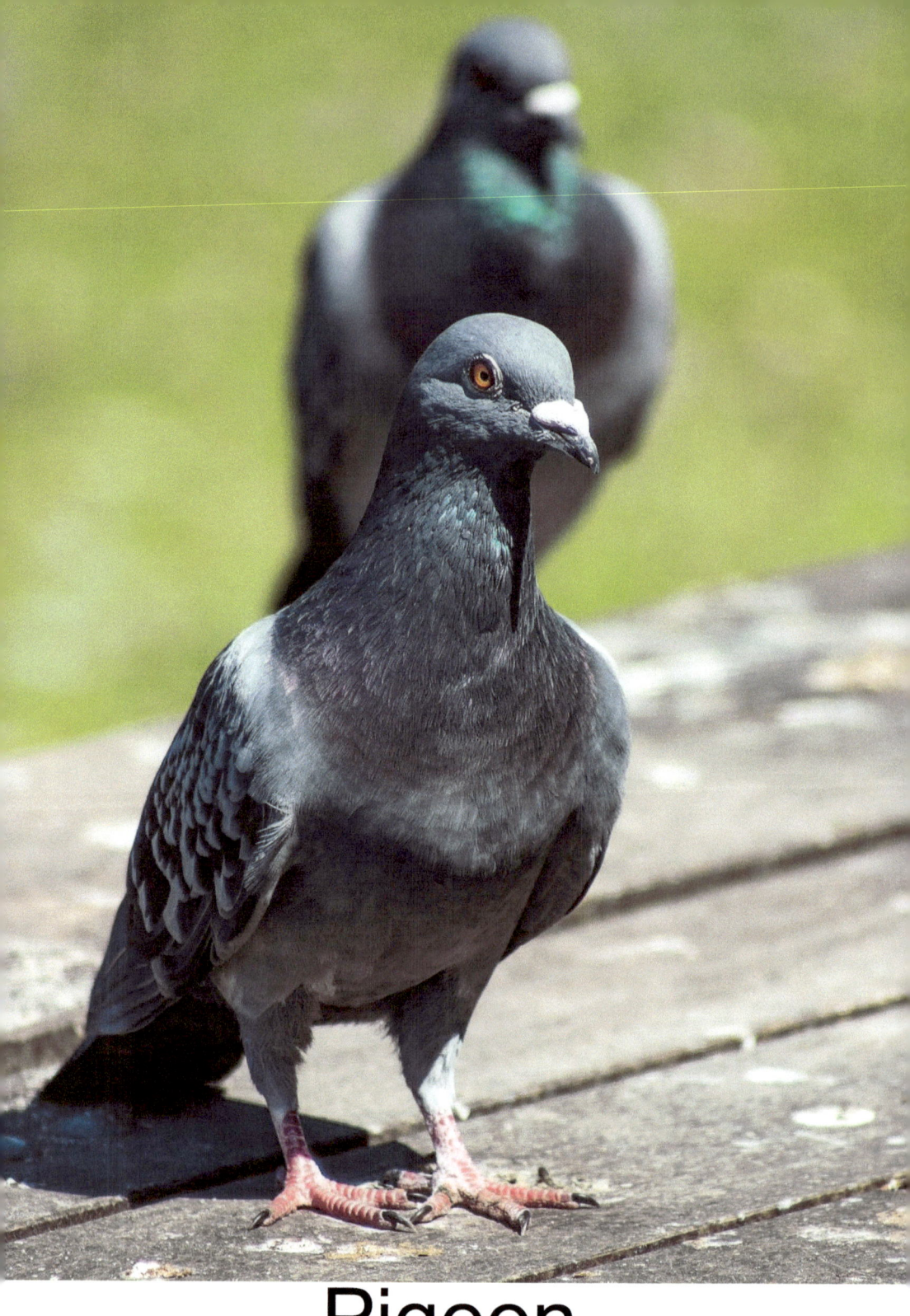

Pigeon

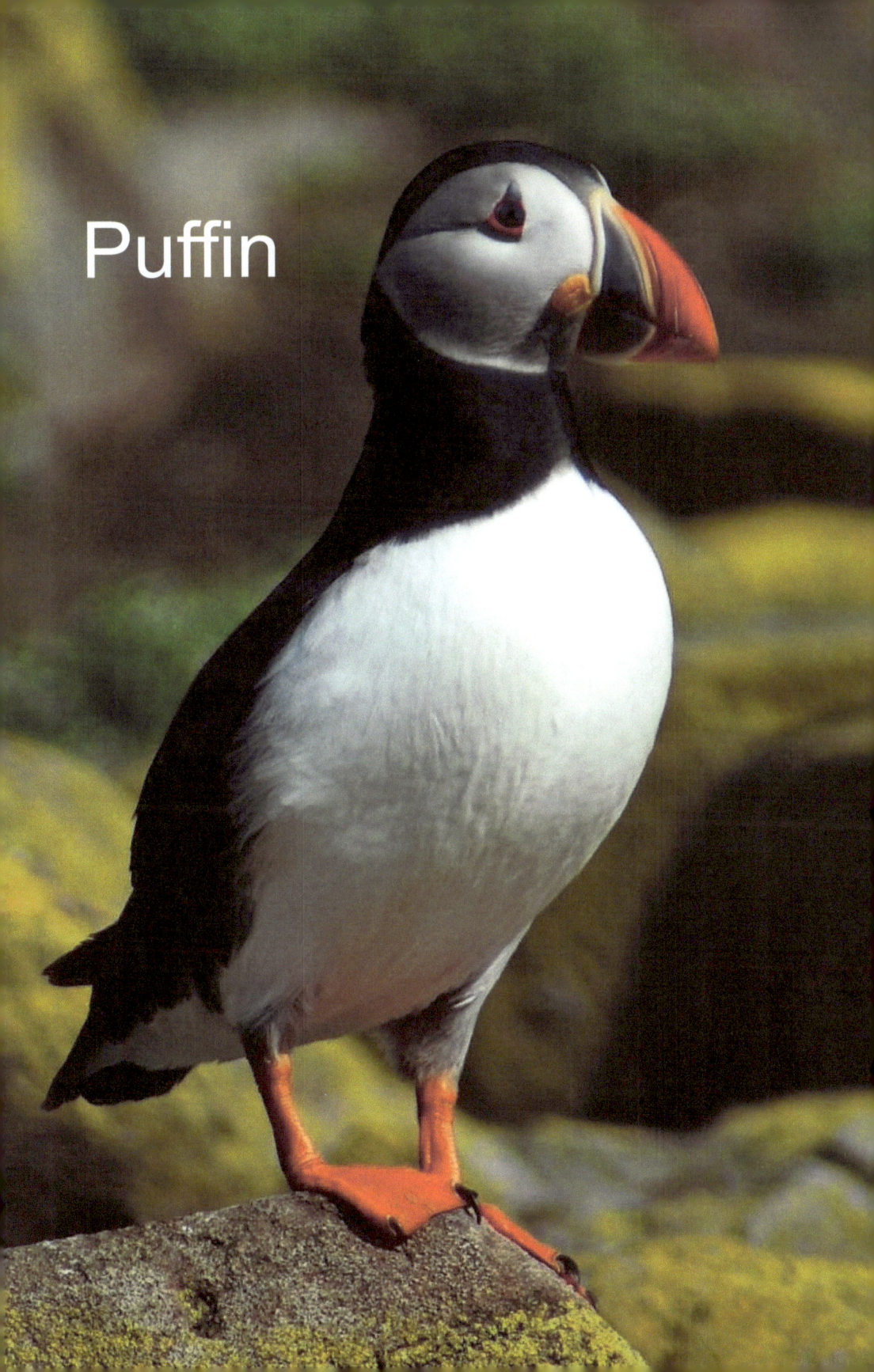

Puffin

River Tern

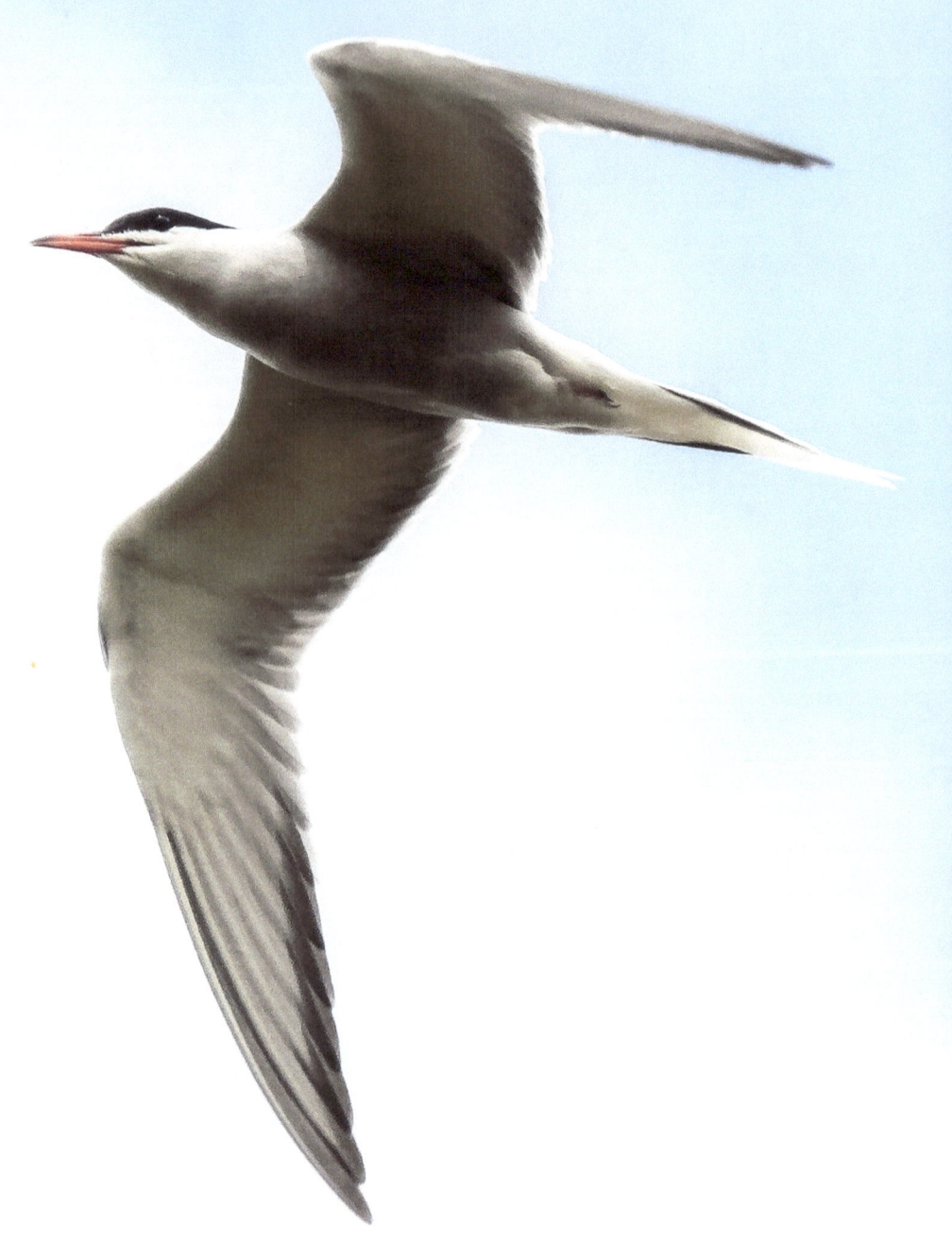

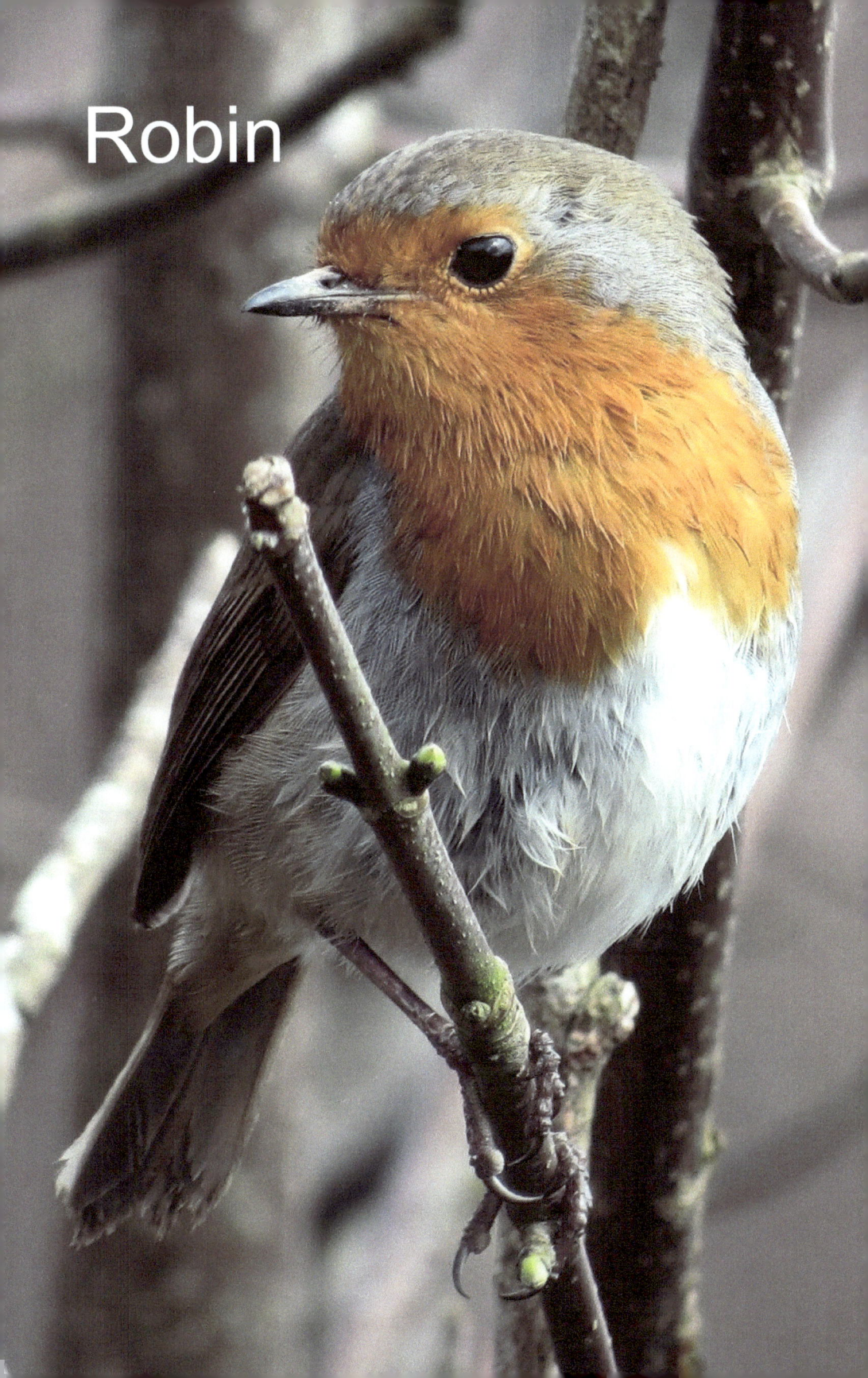

Robin

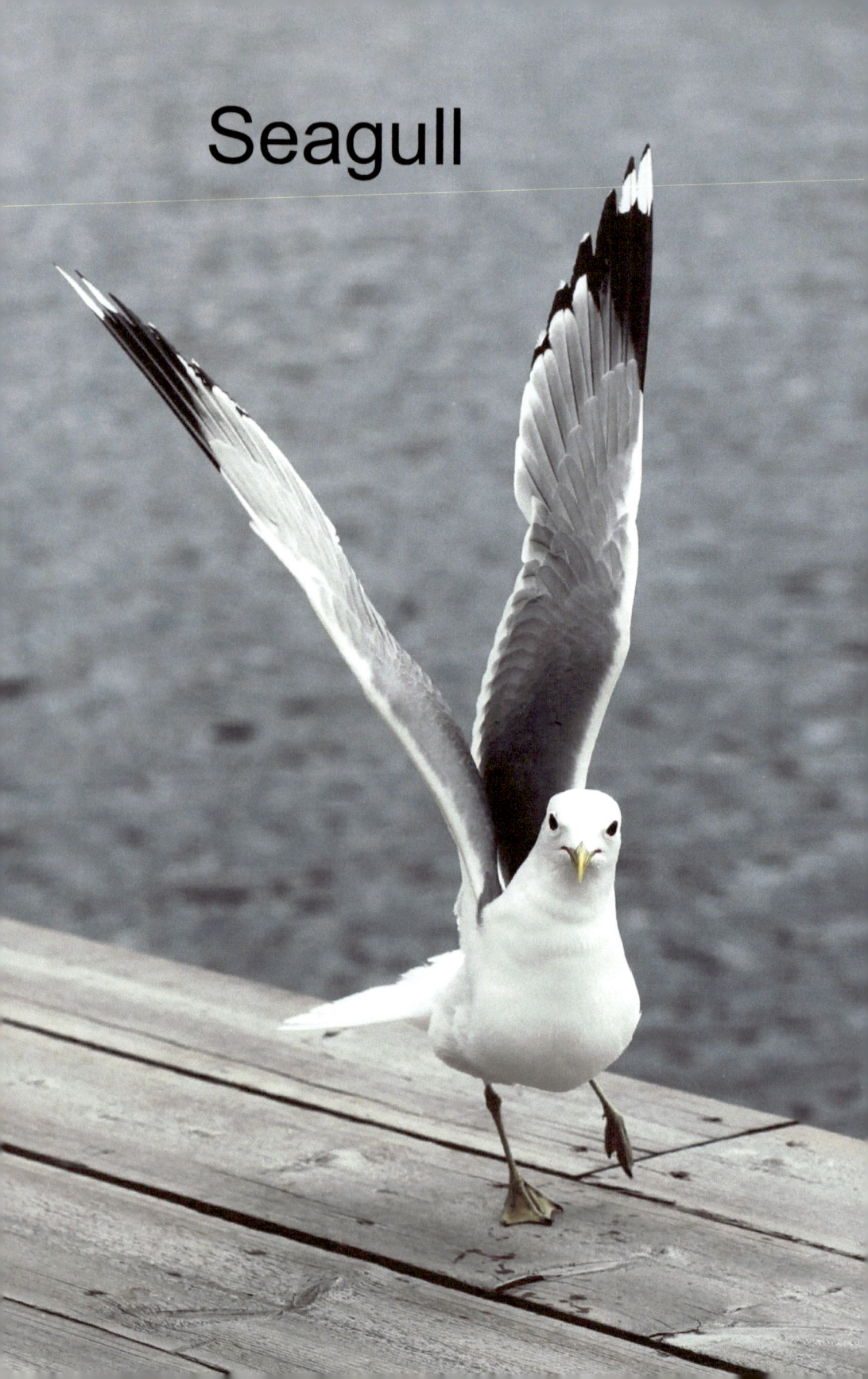

Seagull

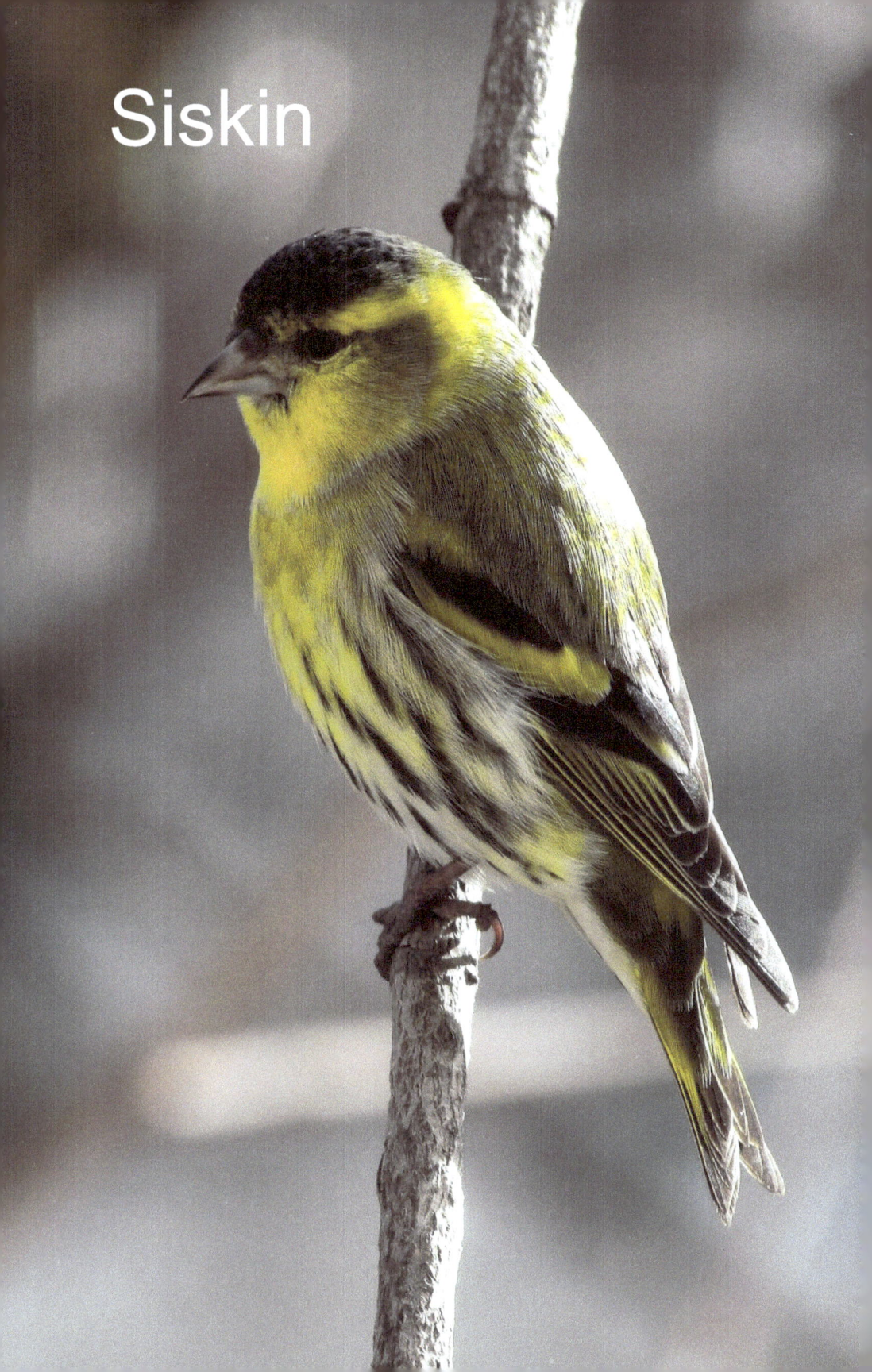

Siskin

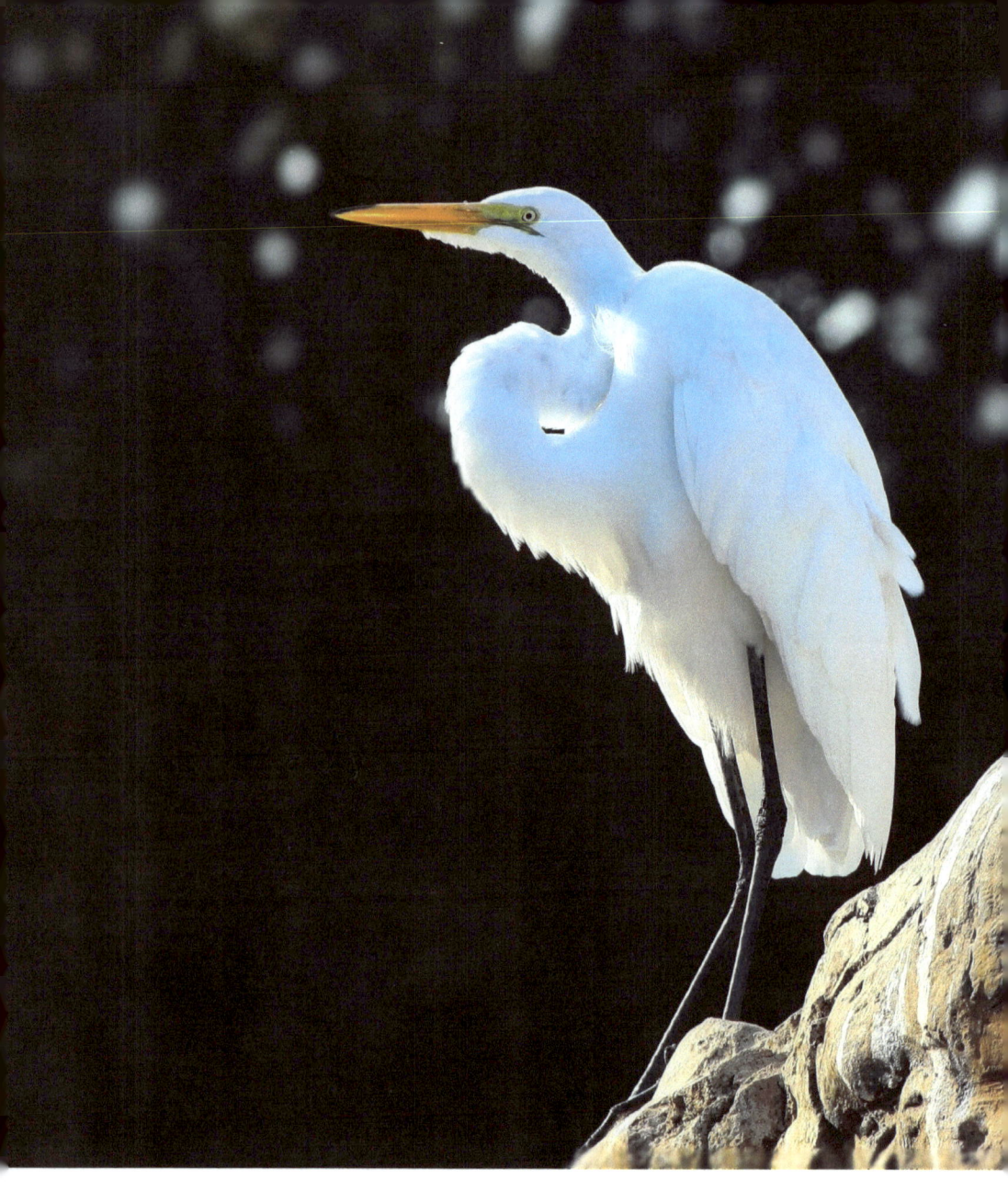

Snowy Egret

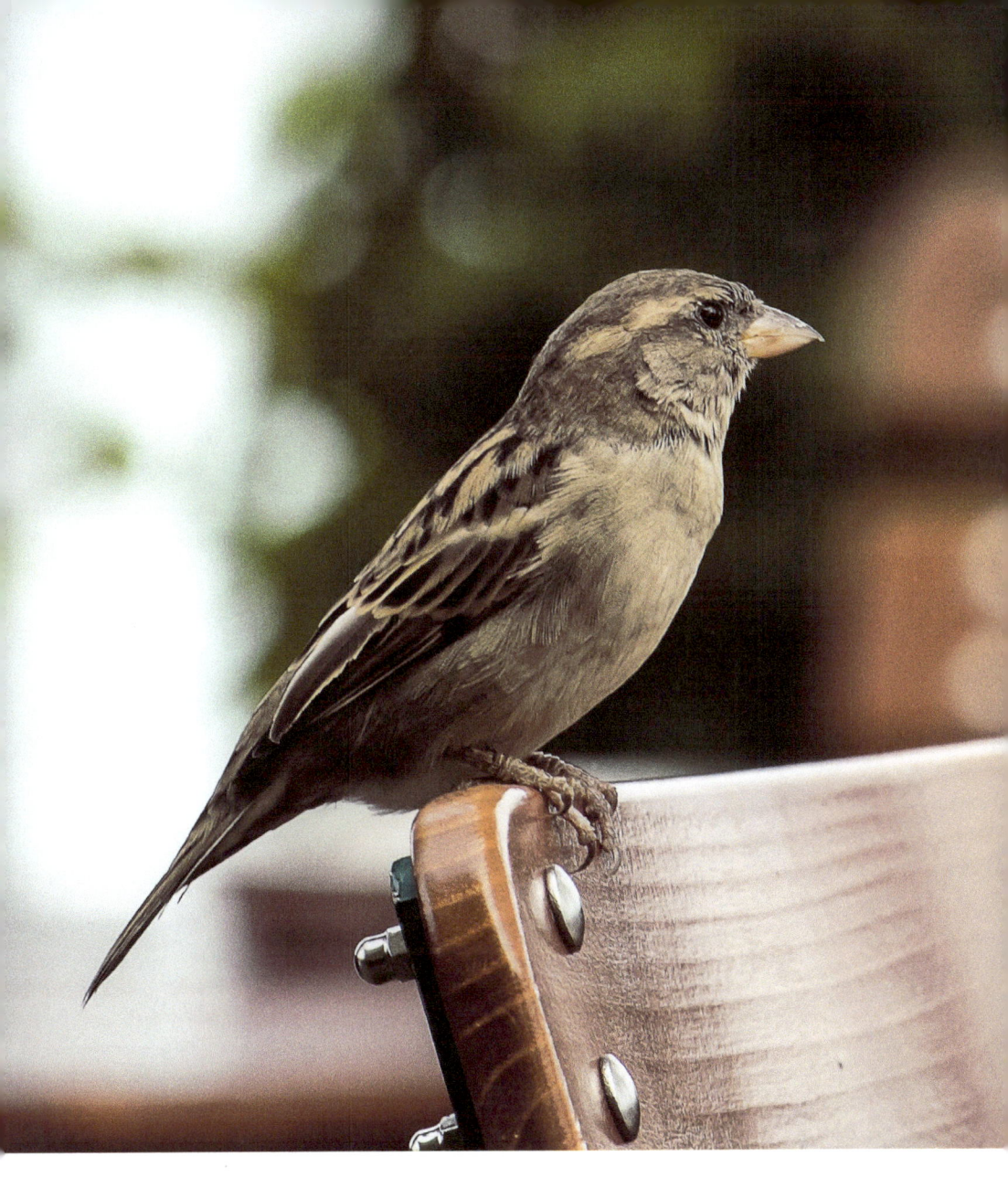

Sparrow

Swan

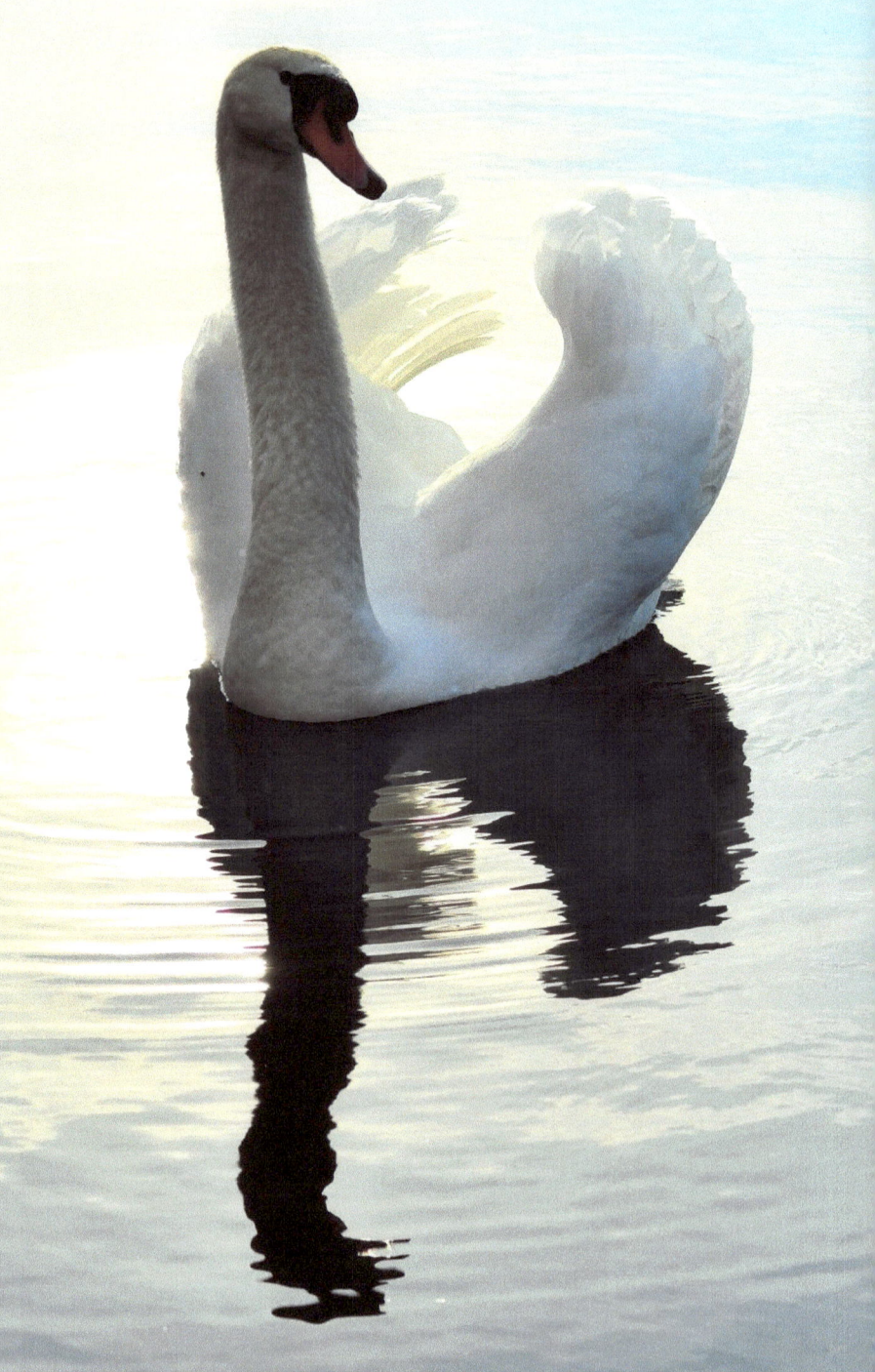

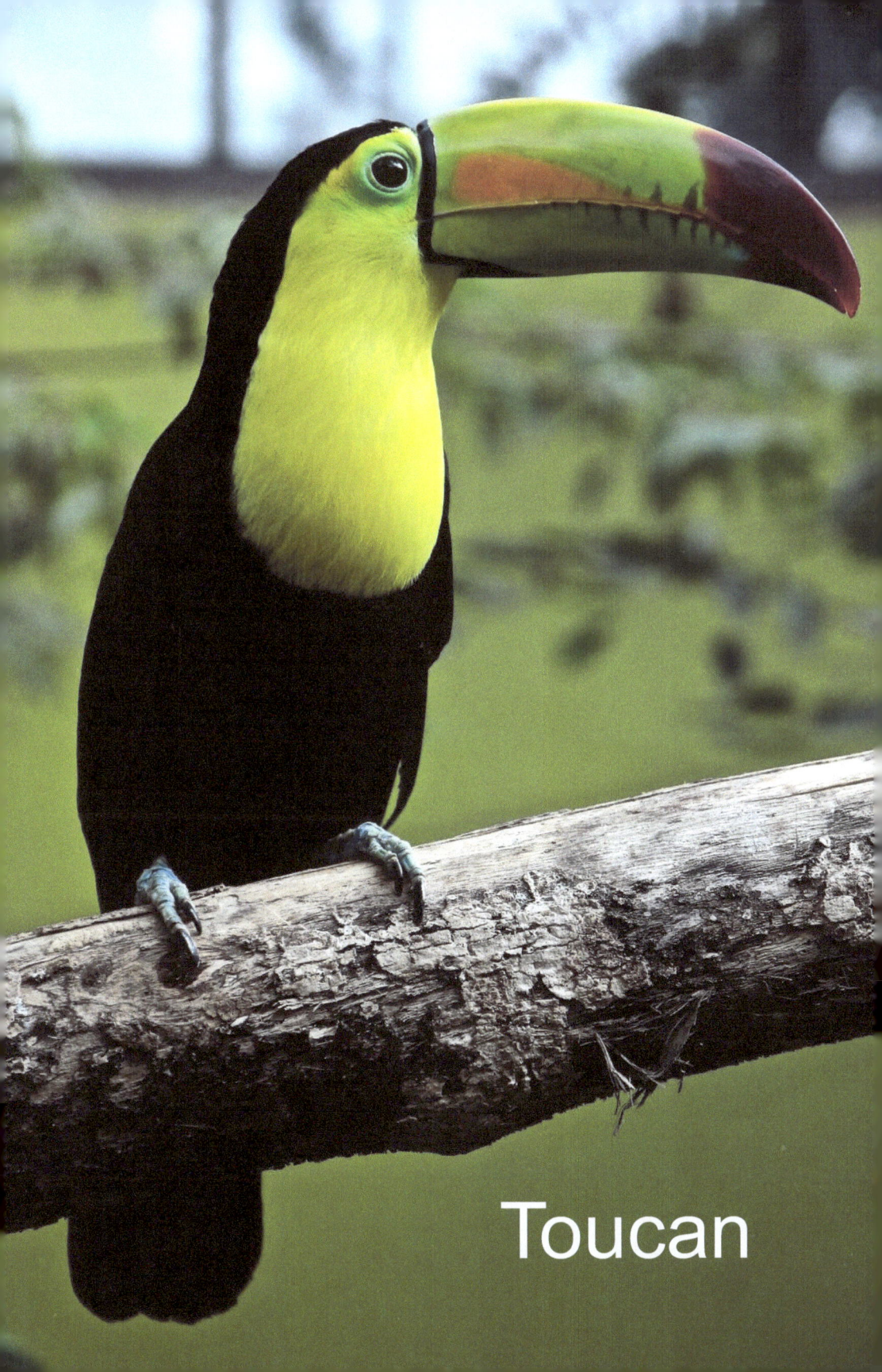

Toucan

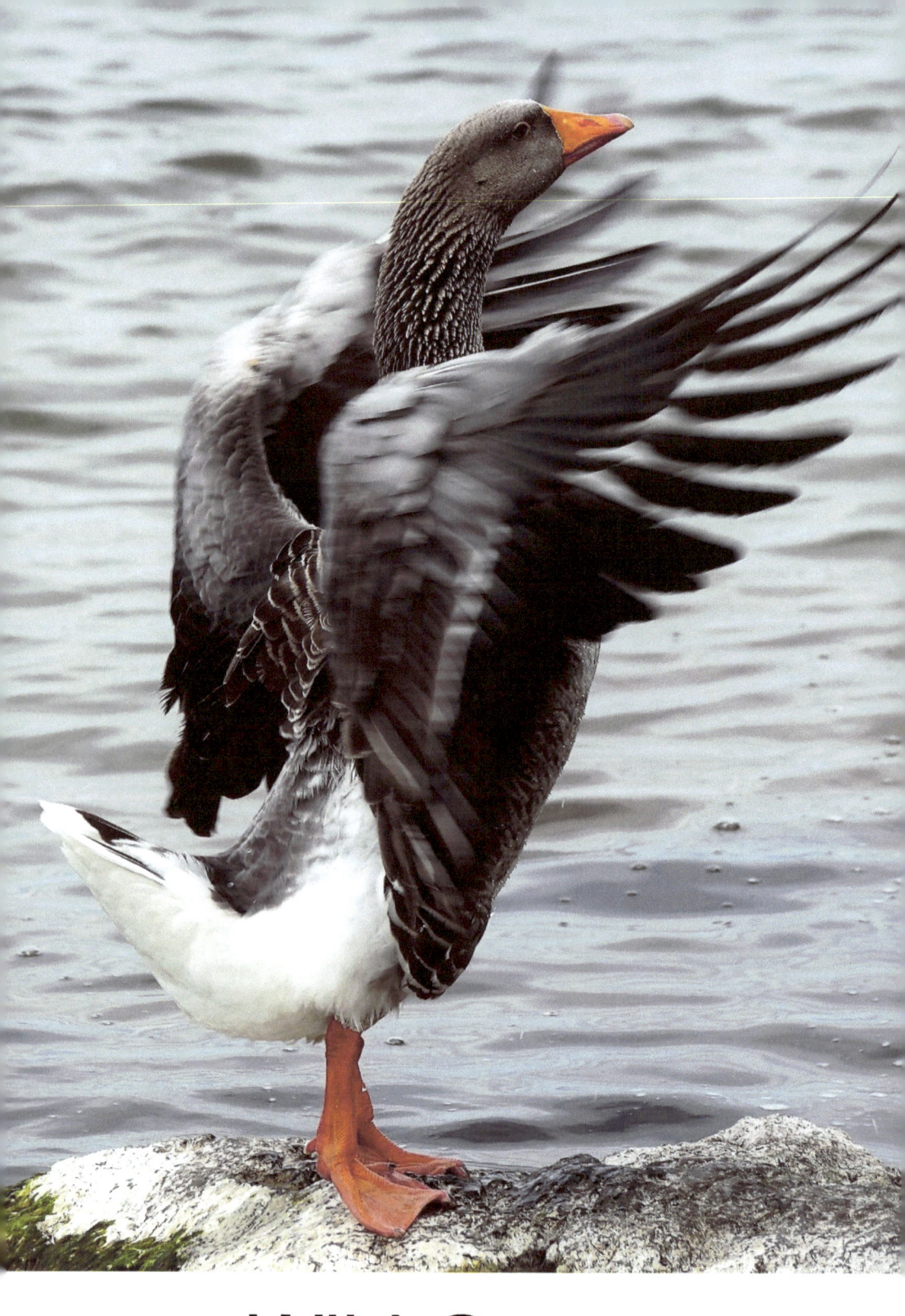

Wild Goose

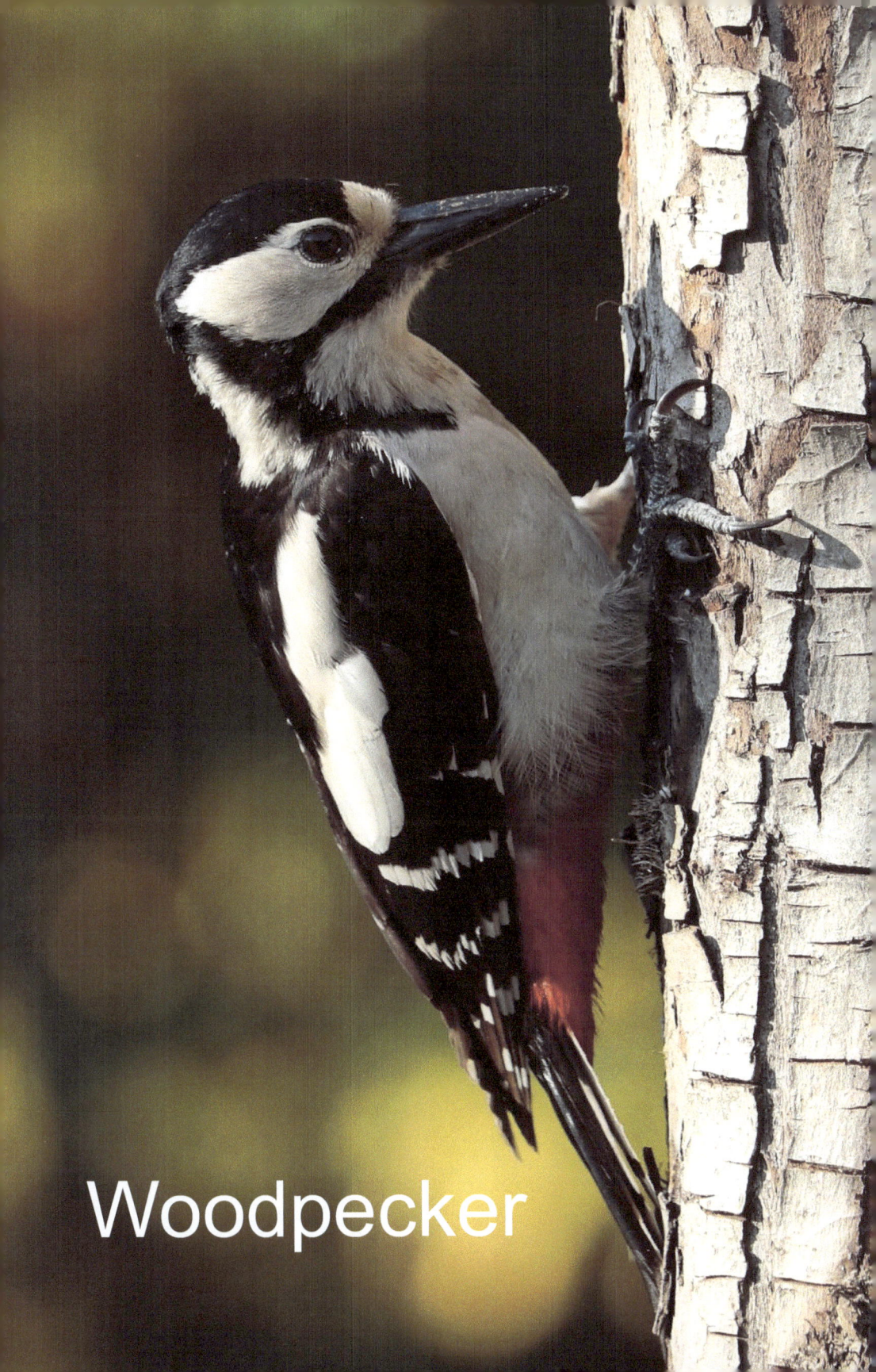

Woodpecker

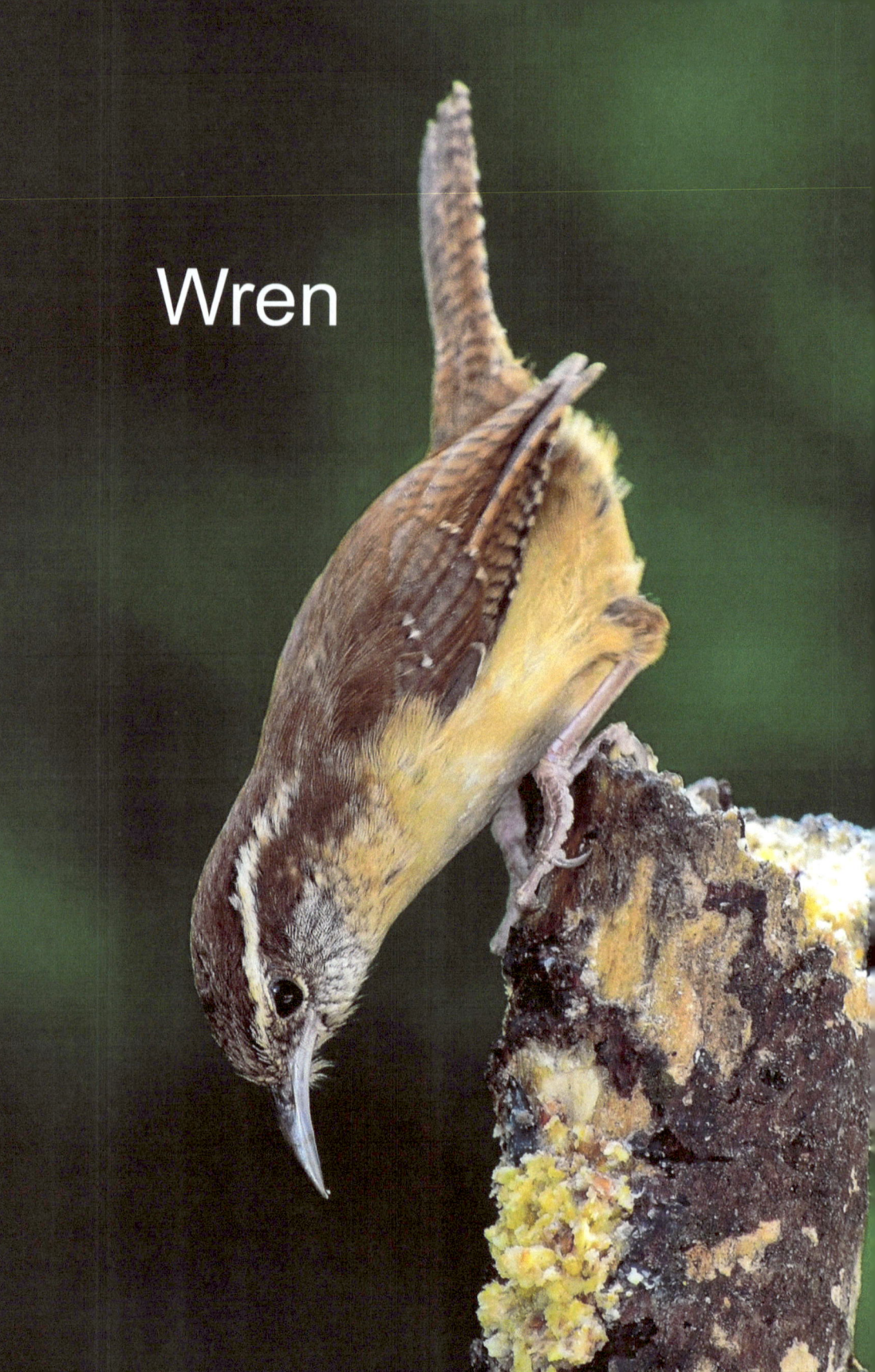

Wren